211493310

EART FAILURE

SUSAN ELLIOT WRIGHT

Type
husband have ____ she is
taking a Master's degree in writing and hopes to divide her
energies between fiction and non-fiction.

Overcoming Common Problems Series

Selected titles

A full list of titles is available from Sheldon Press,
36 Causton Street, London SW1P 4ST and on our website at
www.sheldonpress.co.uk

Overcoming Common Problems

Living with Heart Failure

Susan Elliot-Wright

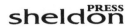

First published in Great Britain in 2006

Sheldon Press
36 Causton Street
London SW1P 4ST

Copyright © Susan Elliot-Wright 2006

The author and publisher have made every effort to ensure
that the external website and email addresses included in this book are
correct and up to date at the time of going to press. The author
and publisher are not responsible for the content, quality or
continuing accessibility of the sites.

British Library Cataloguing-in-Publication Data

A catalogue record for this book is available from the British Library

ISBN-13: 978–0–85969–983–9
ISBN-10: 0–85969–983–8

1 3 5 7 9 10 8 6 4 2

Typeset by Deltatype Limited, Birkenhead, Merseyside
Printed in Great Britain by Ashford Colour Press

Contents

Acknowledgements

I would like to thank all those who were kind enough to share with me their experiences of living with their own or their partner's heart failure, and also those individuals and organizations who helped me to get my facts straight, in particular the British Heart Foundation, who patiently answered my many, many questions.

Introduction

If you're reading this book, the chances are that you, or someone close to you, has been diagnosed with heart failure. If the diagnosis is recent, you're probably feeling quite frightened at the moment – after all, 'failure' suggests that something has stopped working all together. This is not the case with heart failure. Nor is heart failure the same as a heart attack, although if you have had a heart attack, you are more likely to develop heart failure in the future.

Heart failure is the term used to describe a heart that is losing its pumping efficiency. It can affect the left side of the heart, the right side, or both sides, and can cause symptoms such as breathlessness, lack of energy, swollen ankles and a general feeling of being unwell. Although heart failure affects both men and women, men are at slightly higher risk than women, reflecting the fact that heart attacks and angina, which can lead to heart failure, are slightly more common in men.

According to recent surveys, there are currently around 900,000 people living with heart failure in the UK, a staggering 14 million across Europe and around 5 million in the USA. Because heart failure is more common in older people, experts expect these figures to rise significantly in the coming decades, partly owing to an ever-growing ageing population but also, more alarmingly, to widespread ignorance about the condition. A survey by SHAPE (Study of Heart Failure Awareness and Perception in Europe), published in 2005, found that, even though over 90 per cent of the 8,000 people surveyed had heard of heart failure, only 3 per cent could identify the typical symptoms. Around a third thought, incorrectly, that heart failure was a normal consequence of growing older, and around the same number, also mistakenly, thought that modern drugs could not prevent the condition. Many people, it seems, don't understand what heart failure is, which – given the rather misleading name of the condition – is understandable. Researcher on the SHAPE study, Professor William Remme, was concerned that lack of awareness about heart failure meant that people suffering from it may not seek medical help quickly enough and were 'also unlikely to demand appropriate measures from health-care providers'. He also stated that 'ignorance of the symptoms and of what can be done to treat and prevent the condition could contribute to unnecessarily poor quality of life in tens of thousands of patients and thousands of premature deaths . . .' See http://www.shapestudy.info/ for more information about the SHAPE study.

If you or your loved one has been diagnosed with heart failure, your mind will probably be buzzing with questions and, even if your doctor or specialist has explained the situation in detail, you may well find that you haven't taken very much in. This book aims to address some of these questions, to explain what's happening to you in a straightforward and easy-to-understand way, and to give you information, help and advice on what treatments may be available and what you can do to help yourself. Chapter 3 looks at the process of diagnosis and, briefly, at how actually receiving your diagnosis might affect you – a subject that is gone into in more depth in Chapter 7, which discusses anxiety, depression and stress along with suggestions for coping.

As you're reading this book, you're probably one of the many people who feel that learning as much as they possibly can about the condition that affects them actually helps in coming to terms with it. In learning about heart failure, you first need to know roughly how a normal, healthy heart works and what its precise function is within the body. This is looked at – without being too technical – in Chapter 1. As you'll see from this chapter, the heart is a wonderfully designed component of the incredible machine that is the human body. But like all wonderfully designed components, it can go wrong or simply wear out, sometimes leading to heart failure. In a few cases, heart failure is the result of a viral infection or a congenital heart defect – an abnormality of the heart that has been present since birth. Chapter 2 looks at the more common causes of heart failure and who is likely to be most at risk.

One of the most important questions after a diagnosis of heart failure is: what can be done? The short answer is: a lot! While heart failure can't be 'cured', in that a damaged heart muscle will always be damaged, it is certainly possible to treat the symptoms and to prevent or reduce further damage. It is also often possible to treat the underlying cause of the heart failure. There are a number of drug treatments that have proved extremely successful for heart failure patients, prolonging life, reducing hospital admissions and generally

increasing the quality of life for many people. Surgery may also be an option, ranging from fairly straightforward procedures to, in a very few suitable cases, heart transplant. Treatment options are discussed in Chapters 4 and 5.

You'll be pleased to know that there's also a lot you can do on a daily basis to help relieve your symptoms and to prevent your condition from worsening. Chapter 6 is packed with information on how to make changes to your diet and lifestyle that can not only help your condition but will also improve your overall health and fitness, giving you more strength to cope with your heart failure and more zest for daily life.

Having a chronic condition such as heart failure will undoubtedly have a major impact on your life. Chapters 8 and 9 look at some of the practical, emotional and psychological difficulties you may experience; these may include limited ability to carry out day-to-day tasks, sexual difficulties and financial worries, especially if you have to give up your job or reduce your working hours.

If you care for someone who has heart failure, whether that person needs a high level of care or simply wants someone to talk to about the condition and to share the burden in general, you will have questions, worries and needs of your own. Chapter 10 aims to look at heart failure from the perspective of the carer and to address some of the concerns you may have.

Heart failure can be very mild, or it can be very severe, and being diagnosed with this condition can be very frightening indeed. But try to remember that large numbers of heart failure patients go on to live active and fulfilling lives for many years after their diagnosis, often enjoying better health than they did before! The more you understand about your condition and its treatment, the less scary it will seem, but the workings (and non-workings) of the human body are complex, and with the best will in the world busy doctors may not have time to explain things fully. This book aims to help fill in the gaps and to offer practical suggestions and advice on ways you and your loved ones can take an active role in managing and improving your condition. If you're newly diagnosed, you may still be feeling quite poorly; however, with treatment from your doctor and changes you can make to your diet and lifestyle, your condition should improve fairly rapidly, and a few months from now you could feel better than you have for years. Good luck!

1

A healthy heart and how it works

As stated in the introduction, heart failure doesn't mean that the heart has 'failed', rather that it is not working as efficiently as it should. In order to understand heart failure properly, it would help to know how the heart is supposed to function when it is working well. We all know that our hearts beat, but not many of us take the time to think about what that actually means. It's a bit like the engine of a car – as long as it starts when we turn the ignition and ticks over when the engine is idling, we tend not to think about *how* it starts, what keeps it ticking over and what actually makes it move.

Blood circulation

Put simply, the human body needs a continuous supply of oxygen in order to keep the tissues alive and the organs functioning. To achieve this, the heart and lungs work together. We breathe air into the lungs, where the oxygen in the air is extracted and passed into the blood. The heart, which is a double pump made of very strong muscle, then pumps blood containing oxygen and other nutrients around the body. The oxygen and other nutrients move from the blood into the body cells, while the waste product carbon dioxide moves from the cells into the blood. The blood is then carried back to the heart, from where it is pumped to the lungs, where the carbon dioxide is removed in order to be expelled as we breathe out. Fresh oxygen from air breathed in is passed into the bloodstream, ready to go back to the heart, where the whole process begins again.

This process of getting oxygenated blood to the tissues and deoxygenated blood containing carbon dioxide away from them is known as circulation, and the heart and network of blood vessels responsible for the process is known as the circulatory system or the cardiovascular system. The circulatory system is often likened to a central heating system in a house, with the boiler representing the heart, water in the system representing the blood and the radiators being like the various parts of the body. Just as water is pumped through pipes around the house into the radiators to supply warmth, blood is pumped through the blood vessels to the body tissues to supply oxygen. As the cooled water in a central heating system returns to the boiler to be reheated, so the blood returns to the heart and lungs to be re-oxygenated.

How does the heart work?

The human heart is about the size of an orange or a small grapefruit and is made up largely of muscle. Heart muscle, known as myocardium (from the Latin *myo*, muscle, and *cardium*, heart) is a particularly strong type of muscle, as considerable power is needed for the heart to pump blood around the body. The heart does this by continuously contracting and relaxing throughout our lives, whatever we're doing and even while we're asleep.

The heart is divided into four hollow chambers, upper chambers, known as atriums or atria, and lower chambers, called ventricles. The upper filling chambers are connected to the lower pumping chambers by valves that stop the blood from flowing in the wrong direction. Similarly, the ventricles are connected to arteries to the lungs and the rest of the body by valves that keep the blood going in the right direction.

What is a heart 'beat'?

Blood from around the body – in other words, blood that has given up its oxygen and now contains carbon dioxide – flows back towards the heart via a network of veins. This network feeds into two very large veins, one called the superior vena cava, which comes in at the top of the right atrium and brings blood from the upper body, and one called the inferior vena cava, which enters from the bottom of the right atrium and brings blood from the lower body. As soon as the relaxed right atrium is full of this deoxygenated blood, it contracts, forcing blood through the tricuspid valve (an inlet valve) into the right pumping chamber, the right ventricle. A split second later, the ventricle contracts, the tricuspid valve closes and the pulmonary valve (an outlet valve) opens to allow the blood to pass into the pulmonary artery. (The word 'pulmonary' means 'to do with the lung'.) The pulmonary artery is a huge blood vessel that divides into two to carry blood to the left and right lungs so that it can dump the carbon dioxide and load up with more oxygen. Once the carbon dioxide has been breathed out, and the blood enriched with fresh oxygen, it flows back via the pulmonary veins to the left atrium or filling chamber. Although blood leaving the heart is sent round the body by means of a powerful pumping mechanism, the process of returning it to the heart is slightly more complicated, involving a combination of gravity (in the case of the upper body), the contraction of certain muscles (especially in the legs) and the action of breathing – as we breathe in, the lungs fill with air, sucking blood up into the chest. When the left atrium is full, the mitral valve opens into the left ventricle where the ventricle contracts, the valve shuts and blood is pumped through an outlet valve – the aortic valve – into the aorta. This is the main artery and the largest blood vessel in the body. The other arteries you might hear about are the coronary arteries which are attached to the surface of the heart and supply the heart muscle itself with the oxygen-rich blood it needs to function efficiently.

This whole process of the heart relaxing (called the diastole phase) and contracting (called the systole phase) is in fact one heartbeat, and the 'lub-dub' sound of a heartbeat is actually the sound of the valves opening and closing. Although it takes a while to describe it, in practice, the two atria actually contract at the same time, as do the two ventricles. A healthy adult heart beats around 70 times a minute, pumping roughly five litres of blood around the body.

What makes the heart keep beating?

In the case of most muscles, movement is the result of an electrical signal or impulse from the brain. For example, you want to drink a cup of tea, so your brain sends 'messages' down the nerves and into the different muscles required to reach out, grip the cup, lift it to your lips, take a sip, swallow the tea, etc, etc. Although this is not a conscious action in that you don't think, 'lift arm, move forward, grip cup', it is conscious in that the contracting and relaxing of the various muscles occurs as the result of thinking, 'I want to drink a cup of tea'. The heart, however, keeps contracting and relaxing right through our lives, even if we're in a coma. Like other muscles, the heart responds to electrical impulses, but it has its own power supply in the form of a sort of natural pacemaker, controlled by the part of the brain responsible for automatic functions such as heart rate, body temperature control and breathing. This pacemaker, called the sinoatrial node, is situated in the right atrium, and it keeps the heartbeat at a regular rate of around 70 beats a minute. It sends out constant electrical impulses that spread through the atria stimulating the heart muscles to contract.

Some parts of the body need different amounts of oxygen at different times, and blood is automatically diverted away from one part of the body in order to deliver more to another part that needs it at the time. For example, if we run up a flight of stairs, blood will be diverted away from the digestive system and towards the limbs so that the muscles involved in running upstairs will have a greater supply of oxygen. Similarly, if we've just eaten a meal, more blood is pumped to the stomach and intestines in order to help them with the arduous task of breaking down the food we've eaten into the various nutrients and waste products so that they can be utilized or disposed of according to the body's needs. Using the central heating analogy again, we could say that the way in which the body sends more blood to the limbs when we're running upstairs is similar to the way you can turn up a thermostat on a radiator when you want the room you're using at the time to be warmer than those you're not using.

Your pulse

In order to tell how fast your heart is beating, a doctor or nurse will 'take your pulse'. The pulse is simply the wave created by the contraction of the heart muscle, rather like the ripples from a stone dropped into a pond or the waves that wash ashore when a motor boat moves along on the river. You've probably felt your own pulse by placing one thumb on your inner wrist just below the base of the other thumb, and you may have wondered why you can feel it in your wrist. In fact, a pulse can often be felt at several points in the body where the arteries are near the surface. For example, you can feel a pulse on either side of the neck from the carotid artery, or in the fold of the groin from the femoral artery. Arteries are the blood vessels that take bright red oxygenated blood to the tissues, while veins carry the darker, deoxygenated blood back to the heart from the body.

The heart is a fascinating and complex piece of machinery,

4

designed to beat millions and millions of times (think about it – 70 beats a minute, 60 minutes in an hour, 24 hours in a day and so on). No central heating pump ever worked that hard!

2

What causes heart failure?

What does 'heart failure' actually mean?

The term heart failure, as already stated, is a slightly misleading one. Usually, if we say something 'failed', we mean it didn't work or it stopped working. This is not the case with the heart. Heart failure is diagnosed when the heart no longer works as efficiently as it should, causing symptoms such as breathlessness, extreme tiredness and swelling of the ankles and feet. As we have seen, the heart beats over a hundred thousand times a day. When you consider how many times it beats over the average lifetime, it is not surprising that it can lose some of its efficiency as we get older. This may be as a result of gradual damage, such as that caused by the heart having to work harder as a result of high blood pressure (hypertension), or of sudden damage, such as that caused by a heart attack (also known as a myocardial infarction).

How the body reacts to a damaged heart

When the body realizes that the heart is not pumping properly, it tries to compensate in order to ensure that the body still receives the necessary oxygen. The body's emergency response is to release certain hormones, such as adrenalin. You may have heard hormones referred to as 'chemical messengers'. In the case of adrenalin, the message is, 'We need more blood over here! Beat faster!' Adrenalin is also released when we exercise, or in order to prepare the body for exercise. If, for example, our ancestors were being stalked by a lion, or if we're being followed down a dark alley by a mad axe man, our body needs to make sure we can either slay the lion (or axe man) or run fast enough to get away – this is known as the 'fight or flight' response. Either way, the body tissues would need an extra supply of oxygen for this to work. So when adrenalin is released, whether in response to a night at the gym, a stalking lion or reduced oxygen supply caused by narrowed arteries, the heart receives the message 'more blood needed' and starts pumping harder and faster in order to meet the demand. Initially, this helps – the tissues receive the oxygen they need and the body carries on working fairly normally. However, over time, the extra work the heart is doing (that is, pumping with more force and at an increased rate) causes it to weaken and deteriorate further.

Another of the body's responses to heart damage is to reduce the amount of salt and water excreted in the urine by the kidneys. As a result, the body retains fluid, thus increasing the volume of blood circulating around the body. The higher volume of fluid causes the heart muscle to stretch and contract more forcefully in order to increase the pumping ability. Again, this works fine for a while, but as time goes on, some of this excess fluid begins to accumulate in various parts of the body, especially in the feet and legs, causing them to swell. This swelling is known as oedema. Fluid may also begin to collect in the lungs, and if this happens, you are likely to feel short of breath and may even have difficulty breathing, especially when lying down.

Unfortunately, all this extra work that the heart is doing, in order to compensate for the damage it has already experienced, simply leads to more damage. The left ventricle, which is the heart's main pumping chamber, gradually enlarges, allowing it to contract more powerfully in order to pump the increased volume of blood around the body. Over time, the muscle fibres begin to stretch, leaving the ventricle larger and weaker, and unable to pump effectively. This is known as left ventricle dysfunction.

Thus, while the body copes initially with damage to the heart, the damage actually worsens over time. This is why heart failure is known as a progressive illness, meaning it gets worse as time goes on. It is important that heart failure is diagnosed and treated as soon as possible – it cannot be cured, but the progression can be slowed down, symptoms reduced and further damage prevented.

What causes heart failure?

The most common cause of heart failure is coronary heart disease – in other words, a heart attack or angina (intermittent chest pain, especially after exertion and usually lasting only a few minutes). Coronary heart disease is often the result of hardening and narrowing of the arteries caused by a build-up over time of cholesterol deposits on the arterial walls, a process known as atherosclerosis. If a blood clot forms in a narrowed coronary artery, it will reduce the amount of blood being delivered to the heart and, as a result of the inadequate oxygen supply, the heart will work less efficiently. In some cases, the arteries become blocked, completely cutting off the supply of blood and oxygen to the heart and resulting in part of the heart muscle being damaged. For many people, the heart attack causes minimal damage and the person recovers swiftly. But for others, the damage is significant, increasing the risk of heart failure developing in the future. There are a number of other causes of damage leading to heart failure (see the next section), and the greater the extent of the damage to the heart, the higher the risk of an eventual diagnosis of heart failure. It's important to establish what has led to the heart failing, so that if there is an underlying cause that can be remedied, this can be treated as quickly as possible, thus hopefully preventing or reducing the extent of any further damage.

Who is most at risk?

Although it can affect anyone, heart failure is a little more common in men than in women. Recent studies suggest that, of around 63,000 new cases each year in the UK, 34,000 are men and 29,000 women. In both men and women, the risk, not surprisingly, increases with age. While around one in 35 people aged 65–74 has heart failure, this rises to one in 15 for those aged 75–84 and to one in seven for those over 85. In terms of prior damage to the heart, the greatest risk factor by far is coronary heart disease, and so it follows that anyone who is at increased risk of developing coronary heart disease is also at increased risk of heart failure. This might include, for example, smokers, heavy drinkers, those who are overweight, people with diabetes and people who are suffering high levels of stress. There are a number of other conditions that can also cause heart failure, and anyone suffering from these conditions will be more at risk. These include:

- Hypertension – when the pressure in the circulatory system is high, the heart has to work harder to ensure that the same amount of blood is being pumped around the body. This extra workload causes the pumping chamber to enlarge so that it can contract more forcefully but, as we have seen, this ultimately leads to overstretched muscle fibres, which are weaker and soon lose their ability to pump efficiently.

9

- Heart rhythm disorders – which occur when the heart beats too fast or too slowly, or when the heartbeat is irregular (this is called an arrhythmia). One type of rhythm disorder is ventricular fibrillation, when the heartbeat is so chaotic that the ventricles quiver instead of contracting normally. As a result, the heart does not pump any blood around the body, which can be fatal.
- Heart valve disease – when all is working properly, the four valves in the heart keep the blood flowing in the right direction. However, these valves can become leaky, causing blood to flow backwards (this is sometimes described as incompetence or regurgitation) or they can become blocked, obstructing the flow of blood between the chambers of the heart (this is known as stenosis). In some cases, both may occur. For example, rheumatic fever can cause parts of the valves to become thickened and distorted. This can make it impossible for the 'doors' on the valves to open fully. It can also prevent them from closing. Whether the heart has to pump blood through narrowed valve openings or whether it has to accommodate extra blood leaking backwards, the result is that it has to work harder to pump the blood around the body, which means that it eventually becomes weaker and less efficient.
- Congenital heart defects – some people are born with abnormalities of the heart which may increase their risk of heart failure. Most congenital heart defects either obstruct blood flow in the heart or cause the blood to flow through the heart abnormally. Sometimes, these abnormalities can be corrected by surgery, and this may improve the heart's efficiency although it will not actually 'cure' heart failure if it has developed.
- Obesity – being very overweight will put a strain on the heart, simply because the body mass is so great that the heart has to pump harder to reach all the body tissues. Also, because those who are overweight are likely to be so because of a high-fat, high-sugar diet, they are also more likely to suffer from hypertension, atherosclerosis and coronary heart disease, putting them at even greater risk of heart failure.
- Cardiomyopathy – this is the term used to describe certain types of damage to the heart where no obvious cause can be identified. You may hear the term 'dilated cardiomyopathy', which means the chambers of the heart are enlarged, 'hypertrophic cardiomyo-

pathy', which means that the heart muscle is much thicker than it should be, or 'restrictive cardiomyopathy', which means the heart muscle is too stiff and cannot relax properly.

There are other possible causes as well – for example, heart failure can be caused by infection, such as rheumatic fever or viral infection, or by long-term alcohol abuse.

Can anything be done to prevent heart failure?

As you are probably already aware, a healthy, low-cholesterol diet, regular exercise and a relatively stress-free existence reduces the risk of conditions, such as hypertension and heart disease, that can lead to heart failure. So, strictly speaking, you can reduce the risk. However, realistically, most of us don't eat the perfect diet, our pattern of exercise is more likely to be sporadic rather than regular, and, these days, who can avoid stress? If you are reading this book, it is likely that you or someone close to you has already been diagnosed with heart failure, and as we have already seen, heart failure cannot be cured as such. However, if it is diagnosed in the early stages, much can be done to prevent it from worsening, and the symptoms can be controlled with medicines, diet and exercise. Many people with heart failure are able to carry on living normal, healthy and active lives with only minor adjustments to the way they live. How your heart failure affects your life and the extent to which you can prevent it from worsening will depend largely on the severity of the condition when it is diagnosed. (See page 22 for how the severity of heart failure is classified.) There are a number of very effective medicines that can be used to treat heart failure and make your life much more comfortable. These are looked at in detail in Chapter 4. Chapter 6 explores what you can do in terms of diet, exercise and lifestyle (and you can do a lot!) to improve your overall health, reduce the severity of your symptoms and lower the risk of your heart failure becoming worse.

3

How heart failure is diagnosed

Symptoms

In order to arrive at a diagnosis of heart failure, your doctor will want to know about your symptoms in detail as well as carrying out a thorough physical examination and probably recommending a number of other tests that you'll need to have done. There are a number of classic symptoms that, together with other risk factors such as age and medical history, would probably lead your doctor to suspect you had heart failure. Let's look first at the most common symptoms.

Severe tiredness

Severe tiredness may be an early symptom of heart failure. You may feel fatigued most of the time, even when sitting or lying down. Even the most minor activity can bring on a tiredness that is absolutely overwhelming, and this can have a serious impact on your daily life. This tiredness may be due to the reduced supply of oxygen to the muscles – if the heart has weakened, it won't be able to pump enough blood to the muscle tissues for them to work effectively.

Shortness of breath

Shortness of breath can be very distressing. In cases of heart failure it is the result of the failure of the left ventricle to pump into the arteries efficiently enough to clear completely. Pressure then builds up in the left atrium as the blood 'queues up' to be pumped around the body. This results in the pressure being transported back into the pulmonary veins, which take blood away from the lungs. When under pressure, the water in blood is forced out, causing water to collect in the air sacs inside the lungs. If this is mild and only a small amount of fluid is present, you may not notice any symptoms (although the congestion would probably show up on a chest X-ray). If it is more severe and there is a significant fluid build-up in the lungs, it will be difficult for you to breathe. You may hear this described as pulmonary oedema ('pulmonary' means 'to do with the lung', 'oedema' means 'fluid').

A good way of understanding this is to imagine the lungs as being like a sponge, with all the little holes representing the air sacs, called alveoli, in the lungs. If the sponge is dry, you can easily squeeze it, forcing air out of the little holes and then watch it quickly fill with air again and spring back into shape. If you then allowed the sponge to fill with water, it would be much more difficult to squeeze out, and would take longer to return to normal.

This is what it is like trying to breathe through waterlogged lungs – possible, but requiring a good deal of effort. Someone with heart failure will often feel unusually breathless after activity, such as walking upstairs, or when lying down flat. The fluid in the lungs can make you cough, and may even wake you up at night, in which case propping yourself up with pillows may help.

Swollen ankles and feet

Heart failure can also cause a build-up of fluid – oedema – in the tissues, and this causes swelling, especially in the ankles and feet. It may also affect the legs, groin and abdomen.

Other symptoms

Other symptoms include a hacking cough, nausea, constipation, poor memory, dizziness and sleep disturbances.

It's important to remember that some of these symptoms may not be due to heart failure. For example, being overweight or simply unfit can cause breathlessness and feeling tired after exertion. Those who are overweight may have swollen ankles even if they don't have heart failure. Ankle swelling can be due to varicose veins, especially in women, and is also a side effect of some medicines. However, these symptoms could indicate heart failure, so your doctor will want to investigate further.

Andy

Andy is 47 and has recently been diagnosed with heart failure. Apart from being a smoker, he has a fairly healthy lifestyle and has always been very fit and healthy, so when he began to suffer ankle swelling and breathlessness around Christmas 2003, neither he nor his doctor thought it was anything serious. The doctor suspected asthma, from which Andy had suffered as a child, and suggested an inhaler for his breathing along with diuretics (water tablets) for his fluid retention. Within a week or so, Andy was back to normal and thought no more of it until the same thing began to happen the following year:

It was just before Christmas 2004 when my ankles started to swell again. I went back to my GP, who gave me the same medicine that I'd had before, only this time it didn't work. I wasn't particularly overweight but I began to get heavier. Not only were my ankles swelling, but my legs and stomach as well. I seemed to be filling up from the feet upwards! I'd just started a new job and really didn't want to go sick, so I put up with it, but I just got worse. I became so short of breath that I could hardly breathe when lying down. I ended up sleeping with three, then four pillows, then sitting in a chair. Eventually, I couldn't sleep at all – my breathing seemed to stop as I dozed off. Foolishly, I tried to diagnose myself by looking it up on the internet – I thought I had sleep apnoea! But that didn't explain the swelling and heaviness. I could barely move. My legs were like concrete – I couldn't climb stairs and I had to lift my legs with my hands to get them in and out of the car. When I went back to my doctor he took one look and said 'you've got heart failure!' He sent me straight to hospital and I was admitted immediately. I didn't really know what heart failure was, but I knew I hadn't had a heart attack, so I wasn't too worried. It sounds silly, but I hadn't really thought of what was happening to me as actual symptoms. It wasn't until they asked me about my 'waterworks' that I realized I'd hardly passed any urine in the last few days. I just hadn't noticed. I was retaining so much fluid by this time that I looked like the Michelin man!

My wife was worried sick and my mum and sister cut short their holiday in Hong Kong. By this time I'd begun to realize that it was quite serious and I was starting to feel frightened, especially as I'd never been in hospital before. They catheterized me straight away to get some of the fluid out, then I was given diuretics and various other drugs and told to drink no more than a litre of fluid a day until my weight came down. The weight just fell off, and after a couple of weeks, I was much better and was discharged from hospital. I've always eaten healthily, but when I came out of hospital I cut down even more on salt, fat and sugar, and within a few months I'd lost 26kg, although most of this was fluid. I still smoke, I'm afraid, but I've cut that down drastically, too. I had to go for regular check-ups for the next few months, and they were constantly rearranging my pills, but I continued to improve. Then last September I went for an angiogram (see page 19) and possibly an angioplasty (see page 36) as well. I was terrified as they took me down to the operating theatre. They were very good and explained everything that was going to happen, but I was still nervous. Then I noticed the doctor had an accent. It turned out he was from Germany and, as I spoke German – I met my wife in Germany when I was in the army there – I was able to chat with him in German throughout the procedure. As a result, I completely forgot about my nervousness and the time just flew – apparently, the procedure took 36 minutes, but it seemed like five!

Happily, they didn't need to do an angioplasty and my heart was looking fairly healthy. After the procedure, they inserted what they call an 'angioplug' into the incision site to stop the bleeding. It's a fairly new technique, apparently, and it means they don't have to apply pressure to the wound afterwards. The plug just dissolves in a while, so I didn't need to go back to have it removed.

It's now almost two years since I was diagnosed, and I'm more or less back to normal. I still have to watch my weight and my fluid intake, but I no longer feel breathless and I feel as fit as I did before I became ill. I've always enjoyed life, but I enjoy it even more now!

Confirming heart failure

Your doctor will need to try and establish whether or not there has been any damage to your heart. This will usually involve checking your blood pressure, listening to your heart to check the rate at which it is beating and whether the rhythm is regular, checking whether there is any fluid in your lungs or in other parts of your body, and carrying out blood tests to check for diabetes, thyroid disease, anaemia or kidney damage.

Doctors may also take a blood sample to test your levels of a hormone called natriuretic peptide. High levels of this hormone are often found in those with damage to the heart because it is released in larger quantities when the left ventricle becomes stretched. If your levels of natriuretic peptide are normal, it is unlikely that there has been any damage to your heart, but high levels indicate that heart failure is likely to be due to the left ventricle becoming stretched.

Testing your heart

If the initial investigations suggest that heart failure is likely, your doctor will want more extensive testing to be carried out. This may take place at your doctor's surgery, or it may be at the hospital. Some of the tests will be to see how your heart is performing, others will be to try to determine the underlying cause of the heart failure and to see whether anything can be done about it. It is sometimes possible to cure the cause of heart failure, even though the heart failure itself cannot be cured.

It is perfectly normal to feel quite anxious about these tests, especially as the equipment used to carry out the testing can look quite frightening, even though the tests themselves are very simple and straightforward. If you do feel nervous or anxious in any way, take your partner or another relative or friend with you on the day – just having someone to chat to while you're waiting can make you feel more relaxed. Depending on which test you're having and where you're having it, it may be possible for the person accompanying you actually to sit with you while you're having the test, although there will be some occasions where the other person will have to wait outside. It may be possible for your companion to come in with you to have a chat with the doctor. When we're feeling anxious or nervous, we are often unable to take in what we're being told, so having someone with you who can not only ask questions but can also remember the answers can be very helpful.

Some of the tests that may be done are described below.

Electrocardiogram (ECG)

An electrocardiogram (usually known as an ECG) measures your heart rate and rhythm by picking up electrical impulses from the heart and recording them on paper so that a doctor can interpret them. The test involves having little sticky patches called electrodes stuck onto your chest, arms and legs. The electrodes are connected to wires linked to a machine that records the electrical signals produced by your heartbeat and shows them on a computer screen. This test takes about five minutes and is in no way uncomfortable; it doesn't do anything *to* your heart, it simply records information *from* it.

An ECG can tell the doctor whether your heart rate and rhythm are normal, and it may help him or her to assess whether there has been any damage to your heart from a past heart attack, perhaps, or from high blood pressure, which could be putting it under strain. But although an ECG can provide a lot of information, it is not a conclusive test. An abnormal ECG reading may not necessarily mean there is anything wrong. Similarly, it is possible to have a perfectly normal ECG even when you do have heart disease, so doctors do not rely on this test alone to diagnose heart failure or to confirm a diagnosis of heart failure.

Chest X-ray

A chest X-ray can show whether your heart is enlarged, and whether your lungs are congested with fluid. Again, while it is useful for your doctor to be able to see your heart and lungs, an X-ray alone is not enough to be sure you have heart failure. It may, of course, show another problem with your lungs that could be causing your symptoms, so it's a good test to have. An X-ray is completely painless and usually only takes a few minutes. The radiographer may want to take X-rays from several different angles, and after he or she has completed taking the X-rays, you'll probably be asked to wait while they check that the images are clear enough and show the whole chest area. The radiographer will not discuss the results with you but will pass the X-rays on to your doctor.

Echocardiogram

An echocardiogram is probably the most reliable and widely used test to confirm a suspicion of heart failure. The test uses sound waves to produce a picture of the structure and movement of your heart. This test is also completely painless but is a very skilled procedure and may take up to an hour. The person carrying out the test places a sound probe on your chest while high frequency sound waves are passed through your skin. When the sound waves reach the different parts of the heart, they bounce back and the probe picks up the echoes. By moving the probe around, a 'picture' of your heart is created on the screen – much like the ultrasound scans a pregnant woman has so that doctors can monitor the unborn baby's development. This test can show the structure of your heart so that the doctor can see whether there is any damage to the heart muscle or valves. It can also show if the valves are working properly and whether your heart is pumping blood efficiently.

Exercise ECG (treadmill exercise stress testing)

An exercise ECG is not usually used to diagnose heart failure, but it can be useful in helping the doctor to assess how serious the heart failure is and can also help in the planning of your treatment. The main advantage of an exercise ECG is that it can identify problems that would not show up if you were just sitting or lying down but are apparent only while you are exercising or immediately after exercise.

The test involves placing sticky electrode patches on your chest and linking you up to the ECG machine in the same way as with an ordinary ECG. The doctor will then ask you to exercise, either on a treadmill or an exercise bike, starting off at a fairly gentle pace. As the test progresses, the doctor will gradually increase the difficulty by increasing the speed or slope on the treadmill, or increasing the resistance on the bike so that it would be like cycling up hill. A doctor will supervise the test and will monitor your ECG readings, blood pressure and breathing at each stage. The doctor will record symptoms such as chest pain or shortness of breath, noting particularly the level of exercise that brings on the symptoms. If you become too uncomfortable, the doctor will stop the test. Otherwise, it usually takes 15 minutes or so. Another recording will be taken after you have stopped exercising.

Lung function testing

You may also be given a lung function test. This is not so much to diagnose heart failure as to rule out other possible causes of symptoms such as chest pain and shortness of breath, which could be due to lung conditions such as bronchitis or emphysema.

Angiogram (cardiac catheterization)

Again, angiography is not usually used to diagnose heart failure, but it may be used to establish the cause of the condition and assess its seriousness. The test involves passing a catheter – a long, flexible and very thin tube – into the heart through a vein or an artery. The staff involved in carrying out your test will be 'gowned up' as though for an operation, because it's important that everything is kept sterile. Most people have the test done as a day case although some people will need to stay in hospital overnight. The catheter is usually inserted by means of a needle through the skin in your groin. You'll be given a local anaesthetic to numb the area where the needle goes in, so the procedure shouldn't cause any pain. Sometimes, doctors decide to insert the catheter through a small incision in your arm – again, you'll have a local anaesthetic for this.

Using an X-ray machine, the doctor will direct the catheter through the blood vessels and into the correct position in the heart. You won't be able to feel the catheter moving around, but you may feel a slight 'jump' or palpitations when the tube touches the wall of the pumping chamber, as this will cause the heart muscle to contract.

A colourless liquid, referred to as a 'dye' because it shows up on X-ray, is put into the catheter so that the doctor can 'take pictures' of what is going on inside your heart. You may feel a slight burning sensation all around the body as this is done – the doctor should warn you what to expect. You may also experience a warm feeling in your groin which can make you think you've wet yourself. Don't worry – you almost certainly haven't! The dye enables the doctor to see how well the heart is pumping, whether there are any areas of the heart that don't move and whether any of the valves are leaking. The doctor will also be able to see whether there is any narrowing in your coronary arteries. You may be asked to hold your breath while the X-ray machine takes a picture, but apart from that, all you'll have to do is lie still. You'll be linked up to an ECG recorder during the procedure and your blood pressure, heart rate and rhythm will be checked continuously.

Cardiac catheterization can take from 20 minutes or so up to an hour. When the test is over, pressure will be applied to your groin for a few minutes to stop the bleeding, or if the catheter was inserted through your arm, you'll have a few stitches. You'll then be taken to a recovery area where you can just rest for a while. Many people find they feel absolutely wiped out by the test and need to have a sleep afterwards. A nurse will pop in every now and then to check your pulse and blood pressure and to make sure the bleeding has stopped. If all is well, you'll be allowed to go home the same day.

You may feel a little uncomfortable in the groin or arm as the anaesthetic wears off, and you may find that the site is tender for a while, but most people will be back to normal within a day or two.

Although the test is generally very safe, a small minority of patients do experience problems after it. Serious complications are rare, but they do occur occasionally and could involve the coronary arteries going into spasm or being damaged by the procedure, in which case emergency surgery would be required to carry out coronary artery bypass grafting. There is also a slight risk (between one and two in 1,000) of a patient having a 'serious event' (such as a heart attack or stroke) during an angiogram. No procedure is completely without risk, so this shouldn't alarm you unduly, but it is for this reason that your doctor will not recommend an angiogram unless the benefits are likely to outweigh the (very small) risk.

Other tests

Your doctor may recommend other tests not listed here. If you are unsure what the test you are going to have is for or how it will be carried out, ask a member of your health-care team to explain the procedure.

How serious is heart failure?

It would be disingenuous to pretend that heart failure is a minor problem. However, there are degrees of severity, and many people with heart failure will live a full and active life for many years after diagnosis. Clearly, the less severe the heart failure at diagnosis, the better the outlook, although much will depend on how your treatment is managed and what steps you take to improve your own health. This book looks in detail at what you can do to help yourself in Chapter 6. The main thing to bear in mind is that you will almost certainly be able to make small (or big!) changes to your diet and lifestyle that will reduce the severity of your symptoms and the risk of your condition becoming worse.

How severe is your condition?

People with heart failure can be mildly poorly or desperately ill, depending on how severe their condition is. Most doctors classify the severity of their patients' heart disease using a system devised by the New York Heart Association.

The New York Heart Association Classification of Heart Failure

The New York Heart Association (NYHA) classification has four classes of severity:

- Class I – ordinary physical exercise does not cause undue fatigue or breathlessness.
- Class II – slight limitation of physical activity: comfortable at rest, but ordinary physical activity, for example minor activities such as climbing a flight of stairs, getting dressed or doing housework, results in fatigue, palpitations or breathlessness.
- Class III – marked limitation of physical activity: comfortable at rest but symptoms such as breathlessness occur when walking on a flat surface.
- Class IV – unable to carry out any physical activity without discomfort: symptoms occur even at rest, with increased discomfort with any physical activity.

Classifying heart failure in this way helps the doctor to decide what treatment would be most appropriate and also allows him or her to monitor your condition, checking to see whether particular symptoms are becoming more or less troublesome. It's important to tell your doctor about any changes in your symptoms so that your treatment can be adjusted accordingly, if necessary. It is perfectly normal for the severity of your symptoms to vary from day to day, but a gradual and persistent worsening of your condition should be noted and addressed.

Reactions to diagnosis

Being told you have a life-threatening condition is very scary, but you may have been feeling quite scared even before your diagnosis, especially if your symptoms meant you felt unable to get your breath, which can be very frightening. In some ways, having a positive diagnosis can actually help. You now have a name for your condition, so you can start finding out about it and taking some control. There is no doubt that understanding what is happening to your body can help you to feel calmer about your condition, and being well informed can help you to get the best from your relationships with the medical staff responsible for your treatment. Many areas now have specially trained heart failure nurses. Heart failure nurses play a significant role in your medical treatment, but they can also provide information and advice on a wide range of topics affecting your condition, so if you have any questions or concerns, the heart failure nurse is often a good first point of contact.

Unfortunately, not all areas have a heart failure nurse, and not all medical staff are easy to communicate with.

Anna

This was a big problem for Anna, now aged 68, who wasn't even told she had heart failure until she was about to have private treatment to have a defibrillator implanted:

They told me that my heart had lost 40 per cent of its muscle, but eventually, even though nobody used the term, I realized that what I had was heart failure. Many of the doctors I came into contact with didn't want to discuss my condition with me, and I found that deeply frustrating; I am an intelligent person and I wanted to know what was happening to my body.

I think my heart problems began years ago, probably due to stress. My job was very stressful – I was a social worker, working with abused children, I'd also been through a stressful divorce and then, five years ago, my son was killed in a car accident. I'd already changed my lifestyle by then and had remarried, very happily this time, but I think the damage was done. Even though my husband, Alan, and I began to enjoy a more relaxed life, eating very healthily and living half the time in England and half the time in the south of France, I had a massive heart attack. I was airlifted to Nice where I underwent an angioplasty. After I came out of hospital, I was sent to a residential rehabilitation centre for a month before coming back to England. I have to say, the treatment I received in France was excellent, and they sent me home with a huge file containing reams of notes and even CDs explaining what had happened and what treatment I'd had. But as far as I know, that file has never been looked at – the consultant I saw here said he couldn't speak French, and he put it aside. Over the next few months, I began to feel more and more ill and breathless. I had pulmonary oedema and then I got pneumonia, but I got myself discharged from hospital early because I was terrified of catching MRSA or something similar – the hospital wasn't very clean. I was taking lots of different drugs but things were just getting worse, and although I wasn't worried about dying – I have strong spiritual beliefs and death holds no fear for me – I have a wonderfully happy marriage and I wanted to live for as long as possible.

That was when Alan started looking on the internet and we found the Manor Hospital in Oxford, where they were carrying out advanced cardiac techniques. We got in touch with them and for the first time, we felt that someone was taking a real interest in me as well as my heart! I had a defibrillator implanted last year and I feel much, much better. I can feel the device, and I can sometimes hear it, which is odd. It's not particularly comfortable, but my quality of life has improved enormously, so I'm delighted. The doctors at the Manor have been marvellous, explaining everything and treating me like a human being rather than simply a 'condition'. I've even been able to discuss problems such as loss of libido. Other doctors have glazed over when I've mentioned it; I'm sure they think I should be past all that – a very ageist assumption, in my opinion. I think we need to challenge these attitudes or another 20 years will pass and things still won't have improved. We need to keep asking questions, reminding doctors that we're human beings, just like them.

Anna's operation was carried out at the ExtraLife Centre based at the Manor Hospital in Oxford. For more information on the pioneering work carried out at the centre, have a look at the ExtraLife website or that of the Heart Failure Foundation (see page 106–7).

As we have seen, heart failure can be a serious condition, but there are many different treatment options (which are discussed in the coming chapters) that can help reduce your symptoms and help you to lead a more comfortable and fulfilling life. It may take a while for your diagnosis to sink in, and when it does, you may feel worried and anxious, you may feel angry or you may become depressed. All of these reactions are perfectly normal and, while these feelings may be unpleasant, they will, in most cases, fade and eventually disappear. Not surprisingly, some people with heart failure do become depressed and may need treatment for this as well.

Coming to terms with your diagnosis may not be easy, but there are things you can do that will help. Coming to terms with the diagnosis, and reactions to it, are looked at much more fully in Chapter 7.

4

What can be done to help?

As we have already seen, heart failure cannot actually be cured, but the symptoms usually respond well to medication and much can be done to improve your quality of life as well as to prevent your condition from worsening. Treatment will probably involve a combination of lifestyle changes on your part (see Chapter 6) and the prescribing of certain drugs on the part of your doctor. In some cases, surgery may be recommended, and the surgical options are discussed in Chapter 5. Part of your treatment may involve treating the underlying cause of your heart failure as well as the ongoing condition.

Medicines for heart failure

You will probably be given a number of different drugs to treat your heart failure and problems associated with it, each one having a separate role to play in your treatment. Some people will need to take more medicines than others, but most people with heart failure will need to take a diuretic and an angiotensin-converting enzyme (ACE) inhibitor. Many will also need a beta-blocker, and an anticoagulant and an anti-platelet drug to reduce the risk of blood clots. Like all medications, some of these drugs will cause side effects in some patients. These may be mild or could be quite troublesome. Always tell your doctor if you notice any side effects or changes in your symptoms, especially when starting on a drug you haven't taken before. If you notice a severe reaction, you should seek medical advice immediately. You should also check with your doctor or pharmacist before taking any other medicines, including non-prescription drugs and herbal remedies. And don't be afraid to remind your doctor about any other prescription drugs you are taking – different medicines, including herbal medicines, could affect the action of your heart medicine.

If the side effects are troubling, your doctor may try giving you a different medicine or a different brand of the same drug. When you collect your prescription, you should find the name of the drug on the bottle or pack, but there may be different brands of the same drug, so you may see a generic name (the name of the actual drug) and a brand name on your medicines. If you don't recognize the names of the drugs mentioned in this book, it may be because brand names haven't been included for all of them. So, what is your doctor likely to prescribe, and what side effects might you experience?

Diuretics

Diuretics are usually one of the first drugs given to people with heart failure who have oedema (fluid retention). In an emergency, they can be given by injection straight into a vein, but they are usually taken by mouth in the form of tablets. Diuretics work by causing the kidneys to make more urine, thus removing excess salts and water from the body. This will reduce the swelling in your legs and ankles and should also relieve breathlessness caused by fluid in your lungs. Diuretics also help to reduce blood pressure, thereby reducing the amount of work the heart has to do. You'll probably be advised to try and reduce the amount of salt in your diet (see page 49 for tips) because too much salt can reduce the efficiency of the drug.

Some diuretics may cause you to lose potassium, so you will have regular blood tests to keep an eye on your potassium levels. Low potassium levels can cause abnormal heart rhythms, so if your levels fall, you may be given potassium supplements or you may be put on a 'potassium-sparing' diuretic. Diuretics can also raise your blood sugar levels. This can be a problem if you have diabetes, so talk to your doctor about this.

Commonly used diuretics include bendroflumethiazide, bumetanide, frusemide and amiloride.

Possible side effects include leg cramps, light-headedness, rash, tenderness and swelling of breast tissue. Some of the stronger diuretics act very quickly and you may need to pass urine suddenly and urgently.

ACE inhibitors

When you have heart failure, your body produces a chemical called angiotensin along with an angiotensin-converting enzyme (commonly known as ACE). This enzyme converts angiotensin-1 to angiotensin-2, a substance that promotes retention of fluid and causes your blood vessels to contract, making it even harder for your heart to pump blood around your body. ACE inhibitors work by blocking the action of the enzyme so that the blood vessels relax and widen, making it easier for the blood to flow through them and reducing blood pressure, thus reducing the strain on the heart. These drugs also stop your body from retaining too much salt and water, thus reducing swelling in your feet and ankles. Your doctor will usually start you on a fairly low dose so that your blood pressure doesn't fall suddenly. ACE inhibitors may increase the amount of potassium in your blood and can affect kidney function, so your doctor will want to test your blood now and again to check on this.

Commonly used ACE inhibitors include captopril, enalapril, ramipril, lisinopril, quinapril, fosinopril and perindopril.

Possible side effects include a persistent, irritating, dry cough; skin rashes; and dizziness or fainting – people with heart failure may experience dizziness even if they're not being treated with ACE inhibitors, but you should tell your doctor if this happens because it may indicate a sudden fall in blood pressure. ACE inhibitors can lead to high potassium levels, and you should tell your doctor if you experience nausea, weakness or diarrhoea, because these symptoms could indicate a high level of potassium. You should tell your doctor straight away if you experience swelling of the face, mouth or lips, sudden breathlessness or a severe rash or itching.

Angiotensin-2 receptor antagonists

Angiotensin-2 receptor antagonists work in a similar way to ACE inhibitors and have similar effects in that they help the blood vessels to open up, reducing blood pressure and helping prevent damage to the heart. They also help to reduce swelling in your feet and ankles by preventing your body from holding on to too much salt and water. Angiotensin-2 receptor antagonists are sometimes prescribed for people who cannot take ACE inhibitors for some reason – for example, if the side effects of ACE inhibitors are too troublesome.

Commonly used angiotensin-2 receptor antagonists include valsartan, eprosartan, candesartan, telmisartan, losartan, irbesartan and olmesartan.

The most common side effect is feeling dizzy because of a fall in blood pressure. You may also experience nausea, weakness or diarrhoea, and if any of these happen you should tell your doctor because it could be a sign that you have too much potassium in your blood. Side effects are usually fewer and milder than with ACE inhibitors.

Beta-blockers

When you have heart failure, your body knows your heart isn't pumping as efficiently as it should and so it tries to compensate by producing chemicals called adrenalin and noradrenalin, which make the heart work harder. These are the chemicals that are released naturally as a response to stress or fear – often called the 'fight or flight' response (see Chapter 2) – or when the body needs to cope with exercise. Although the short-term effect is helpful – the heartbeat becomes stronger and faster – the long-term effect is that the extra strain that is put on the heart can do more damage and cause the condition to worsen. Beta-blockers work by stopping the action of adrenalin and noradrenalin, slowing down the heart and making it beat more gently, thus reducing the overall strain. Beta-blockers will also lower your blood pressure, and it's very important to get the dose right in order to prevent the blood pressure from falling too much and causing other symptoms.

Beta-blockers have proved to be very effective in patients with heart failure, reducing the risk of dying from heart failure and reducing the amount of time patients have had to spend in hospital. You may feel worse when you first start taking them, but this is quite normal and it may take a few months to settle down. If your doctor thinks you'll benefit from taking beta-blockers, he or she will probably start you on a fairly low dose and increase it gradually if there are no problems, checking frequently, until the correct dose is reached.

Commonly used beta-blockers include bisoprolol, carvedilol and metoprolol.

Possible side effects include tiredness, cold hands and feet, disturbed sleep, panic attacks, temporary worsening of symptoms, and low blood pressure, which can cause dizziness. Beta-blockers can also narrow the airways, so you may not be able to take them if you have asthma, bronchitis or other lung problems.

Digoxin

Digoxin (brand name: Lanoxin) is one of the first treatments ever

30

used for heart failure. The drug originally came from an extract of the foxglove plant and was used in the eighteenth century (possibly even earlier) to treat dropsy, the name given in those days to the condition that caused weakness, breathlessness and swelling of the legs and feet. Digoxin works by slowing the heart rate and making the heart beat more efficiently. It is not suitable for everyone who has heart failure, but is often prescribed for people who have abnormal heart rhythms, especially if their heartbeat is fast and irregular. Studies suggest that heart failure in people who take digoxin along with a diuretic and an ACE inhibitor is less likely to get worse and that this combination of medicines may reduce the need to be admitted to hospital.

Possible side effects include abnormal heart rhythms (even though it is often used to treat this!), nausea and vomiting, confusion, and loss of appetite. Digoxin doesn't actually affect the stomach – the nausea, vomiting and loss of appetite are caused by the effect of the drug on parts of the brain.

Spironolactone

When you have heart failure, your body produces an excess of a chemical called aldosterone, which regulates the amounts of salt and water in your body. The excess of aldosterone causes your body to hold on to more salt; it then retains more fluids in order to balance the salt-to-water ratio. Aldosterone also raises your blood pressure and causes your body to release adrenalin and noradrenalin, both of which make your heart beat faster and harder – not good if you have heart failure. Spironolactone (brand name: Aldactone) works by blocking the action of aldosterone, and your doctor may prescribe it if you are already taking an ACE inhibitor or a beta-blocker but are not seeing sufficient improvement in your symptoms. If you have severe heart failure and are already taking an ACE inhibitor, taking spironolactone will probably reduce your risk of dying of heart failure.

Side effects include tender, slightly enlarged breasts in men and diarrhoea. Spironolactone can also affect kidney function in some people.

Anticoagulants

You may be given an anticoagulant if your doctor thinks you may be

31

at risk of developing blood clots, which can cause strokes or heart attacks. When you have heart failure, your blood is pumped around the body more slowly, so there is more time for clots to form. Warfarin (brand name: Coumadin) is a widely used anticoagulant. It works by preventing the production of a protein called fibrin, which helps the blood to thicken into clots inside your blood vessels. Because of their anti-thickening action, anticoagulants can increase the risk of internal and external bleeding, so it's important to get the dose right and to have regular checks to make sure the blood isn't becoming too thin.

There are a lot of other medicines, including non-prescription and herbal medicines that can affect the action of warfarin, so you need to double and treble check with your doctor or pharmacist before taking this drug. You should watch your alcohol consumption as alcohol can increase the affects of warfarin. At the time of writing, people on warfarin are advised not to drink cranberry juice, as this has also been found to increase the potency of warfarin. If you're prescribed warfarin, your clinic should give you an anticoagulant card, which you should carry with you at all times.

Possible side effects include prolonged bleeding from cuts, bleeding that doesn't stop by itself, bleeding gums, severe bruising, blood in the stools (red or black stools), blood in the urine (red or brown urine), and heavier-than-usual periods or other vaginal bleeding.

Anti-platelet drugs

Platelets are small cells in your blood that stick together to form clots when we cut ourselves. Anti-platelet drugs prevent the platelets from sticking together, helping to prevent the blood from clotting and therefore reducing the risk of having a heart attack or a stroke. The best known anti-platelet drug is aspirin, but there are quite a few people who cannot take aspirin because it causes a reaction or affects other conditions they may have, such as stomach problems or asthma. This varies from person to person, so if you're not sure, discuss it with your doctor. If you can't take aspirin, you may be prescribed another anti-platelet drug called clopidogrel (brand name: Plavix).

Possible side effects include indigestion, nausea and vomiting, excess bleeding, and a skin rash. You should tell your doctor straight away if you suffer an asthma attack or have difficulty breathing or if you have swelling of the face or eyelids.

Statins and fibrates

These drugs lower the level of cholesterol in your blood, thus reducing your risk of heart attack or stroke. Most people with heart failure will be given a statin or a fibrate to improve blood cholesterol and triglyceride levels. As well as taking these drugs, however, try to keep active and eat a diet that's low in saturated fats (see Chapter 6).

Commonly used statins include artorvastin, pravastatin, rosuvastin and simvastatin. Commonly used fibrates include bezafibrate and clofibrate.

Possible side effects include stomach upsets, nausea, diarrhoea, constipation and, rarely, muscle pain, cramps or weakness (tell your doctor or nurse immediately if you experience these muscle problems).

Summary

Whatever medicines you are prescribed for your heart failure, it's important to follow the advice of your doctor or heart failure nurse. As with most conditions, there's an element of trial and error in finding the most appropriate treatment for you. You'll be monitored quite closely at first, but it'll be your responsibility to make sure you report any side effects to your doctor and to take your medicines regularly, as prescribed. Heart patients often have to take many different pills, so you may find it helpful to buy a special pill container from the pharmacy that has separate compartments for the days of the week – that way, you can be sure you don't forget your pills or take a double dose. Make sure you request your repeat prescriptions in plenty of time, and if you're going away on holiday, take care to ensure you have enough of your medicine to see you through your stay and over weekends and bank holidays.

5

Could surgery be an option?

For some people with heart failure, surgery or other invasive but non-surgical procedures may be appropriate. Whether or not you are likely to benefit from surgery will depend on several factors, including what is causing your heart failure. If it's due to a damaged or faulty heart valve, for example, it may be possible to repair or replace the valve surgically. If you have angina (chest pain) caused by the blood vessels that supply blood to your heart muscle becoming narrowed, doctors may be able to carry out a procedure to widen them so that blood can flow more freely through these arteries and more oxygen can get to your heart muscle. The other type of surgery available is a heart transplant. This is only offered to a few patients and may be an option if your heart failure is severe and cannot be relieved by drug treatments. Other procedures include the insertion of a pacemaker or defibrillator. These devices may be used if you suffer from a heart rhythm disorder.

Heart valve surgery

As discussed earlier, the valves in your heart are there to make sure that your blood flows through your heart in the right direction. If one of the valves becomes weak or isn't opening or closing properly, the blood can leak backwards into the chambers of the heart instead of being pumped around the body. This means your heart has to work harder, your body tissues don't receive enough oxygen and you begin to suffer the symptoms of heart failure.

Doctors can usually tell if there's a problem with the valves by listening to the sounds your heart makes or by carrying out tests such as an echocardiogram (see Chapter 3). If the valve is leaking but is not seriously damaged, it may be possible for surgeons to repair it. If the damage is too serious to be repaired, it may be able to be replaced, either by a mechanical valve, made of plastic or metal, or by a 'tissue' valve from a human or an animal.

Repair or replacement of the heart valves is major surgery, carried out under a general anaesthetic. To work on your heart, the surgeon needs to open up your chest and cut through the breastbone to get to the heart, then stop it beating while the operation is carried out. Your body still needs a blood supply, though, so you'll be linked up to a heart–lung bypass machine, which diverts the circulation away from the heart and lungs and makes sure the blood is pumped around the body while the surgery is being carried out.

One of the disadvantages of mechanical valves is that they often make a clicking sound. This is quite normal and, although it's a bit odd at first, you'll soon get used to it and it doesn't mean there's a problem with your new valve. There is a slight risk of blood clots developing on the surface of the valve, but to reduce the risk of this happening, you'll probably be given an anticoagulant (blood-thinning) drug such as warfarin (see Chapter 4). If you take warfarin, you'll be monitored at first to make sure you're on the right dose, as too high a dose can lead to bleeding problems. You should always check with your doctor or pharmacist before taking other medications, and make sure you tell your dentist (and any other practitioner treating you) that you're taking warfarin. It's also important to tell practitioners if you have an artificial heart valve.

Both mechanical and tissue valves can wear out, meaning a second replacement is required. In younger, more active people, tissue valves tend to wear out more quickly, which is why they are usually used for older, less active people.

Coronary angioplasty

Coronary angioplasty (also called balloon angioplasty, balloon dilation or PTCA – percutaneous transluminal coronary angioplasty) is a revascularization technique, that is, a treatment for blocked arteries that ensures that they are able to deliver enough oxygen and nutrients to the heart muscle. Revascularization techniques involve either the widening of narrowed arteries or the bypassing of a blocked artery.

The procedure is carried out under a local anaesthetic and you'll probably be able to go home the next day. A long, thin tube (a catheter) with a tiny balloon attached to the end will be inserted through a small incision in your groin or arm. Using an X-ray machine linked to a screen, the operator will guide the catheter through the artery to the narrowed or blocked section. The balloon is then inflated gently so that it flattens the mass of fatty tissue causing the obstruction against the artery wall, thus widening the space through which the blood flows. The catheter contains a short tube of stainless steel mesh called a 'stent', which expands as the balloon is inflated to hold the artery open. The balloon is then deflated and removed, leaving the stent in place.

Not everyone is suitable for angioplasty, and if your doctor thinks you may benefit, you'll probably need to have an angiogram (see Chapter 3). Currently, only around half those tested are suitable; this is because, in many cases, there are too many narrowings in the arteries, or the narrowings are too tight or too long, for the procedure to work. Although it can be a difficult procedure, angioplasty is usually very successful.

Coronary artery bypass

Coronary artery bypass surgery involves a new blood vessel being grafted onto the heart to get around (bypass) the narrowed part of the coronary artery. The operation involves opening up the chest area by cutting through the breastbone. The surgeon will then graft part of a healthy blood vessel from somewhere else in your body, such as your leg, onto your heart between the aorta and a point on the coronary artery beyond the narrowed or obstructed sections. Several blockages can be bypassed during the same operation and, in most cases, the surgeon will carry out three or four grafts in order to make the bypass last as long as possible. Usually, your heart will be stopped during the procedure and a heart–lung bypass machine used to keep your circulation going. Again, this is major surgery, carried out under a general anaesthetic and requiring a stay in hospital of around 7–10 days and a convalescence time of up to six months, depending, of course, on your age and general health.

Most people find this type of surgery improves their angina. However, the operation will not stop atheroma (the build-up of fatty deposits in the arteries) from occurring inside the graft and causing it to narrow or become blocked. Narrowing of the graft happens to around one in 20 patients each year, and is more likely to affect those who continue to smoke or in whom blood pressure and cholesterol levels remain high.

Around 4–6 weeks after your operation, you should be invited to attend a cardiac rehabilitation programme to help you to get back to as normal a life as possible. This usually involves attending sessions once or twice a week for 6–8 weeks or so. The programme usually includes exercise sessions and lots of advice on diet and relaxation techniques.

Heart transplantation

If your heart failure is severe and cannot be controlled by drugs or improved by other surgery, a heart transplant may be a possible option. Although this amazing procedure has improved and become much more common since it was first carried out by Christiaan Barnard in 1967, there are still only around 150 heart transplants each year in the UK. This is partly due to improvements in treatment, partly to the shortage of donor hearts, and partly to the fact that not every patient is suitable for the procedure. At the time of writing, there are around 100 patients on the active waiting list for a heart transplant. Whether you are suitable will depend on a number of factors, such as the presence of other illnesses and whether you are fit enough to undergo the operation and to cope with the difficulties that may arise as a result of it.

If your cardiologist thinks you may be suitable, you will be referred to a transplant centre for a 'transplant assessment', which will involve lots of tests. These may include blood and urine tests, tests to see how well your lungs are working and a number of tests on your heart, some of which you may have had already, such as echocardiogram, electrocardiogram, coronary angiogram and a biopsy.

There is such a shortage of donor hearts that, before you are accepted on to the transplant waiting list, doctors will need to establish that there is a good chance of the operation succeeding. They'll want to be fairly sure that your body will withstand the upheaval of such a major operation, that it will continue to work effectively afterwards and that it will not reject the transplanted heart. Among the factors that will be taken into account are:

- whether you have any other medical condition or infection that could affect your recovery or could increase the risk of complications after the operation;

38

- whether your heart failure has caused damage to your kidneys – the function of all your organs will be checked to see how well they are likely to cope after the transplant, but kidney function is particularly important because damage to the kidneys is a possible side effect of ciclosporin, a drug that helps reduce the likelihood of your body rejecting the new heart; and
- whether the pressure in the pulmonary arteries is too high – heart failure can increase the pressure in the pulmonary arteries (those that lead to the lungs), and whereas your own heart may have adapted to pumping at this higher pressure, a donor heart is less likely to cope; the pressure in your pulmonary artery will be measured during your assessment, and if it is found to be high, you are unlikely to be accepted for a transplant.

The assessment is also the point at which you and your partner or other family member will be able to meet members of the transplant team, which includes a transplant specialist, surgeon, transplant nurses, physiotherapists, psychologists and a transplant co-ordinator. You can ask any questions you have at this stage and if you'd like to talk to someone who has already had a transplant, do ask, as this can probably be arranged and can be very useful.

When a decision has been made, you'll be told whether you are considered suitable or not. If doctors have decided not to recommend you for surgery, it is likely to be because the risks of the operation are too great or because the chances of success are too small. The decision will be fully explained to you, and you'll be able to discuss other options for treatment. In some cases, further investigations will be required before a decision is made. If you are accepted as suitable, you'll either be put straight on the waiting list, in which case you can be called into hospital at any time, or, if the doctor thinks that you're suitable for a transplant but that your heart failure isn't serious enough at this stage, you'll be reviewed regularly and put on the waiting list if your condition worsens.

Transplant and after

The transplant process usually takes around 3–5 hours, after which you'll be put onto a ventilator to help you breathe until you are able to breathe for yourself, which may take a few days. You'll probably stay in hospital for 2–3 weeks after the operation, although some people may need to stay longer.

One of the biggest fears after transplant surgery is that your body will reject the new heart, so you'll need to take drugs to reduce the risk of this happening. Rejection is the most common complication after a heart transplant. Your immune system treats the new heart as foreign tissue and produces antibodies to attack and destroy it. You'll be given a number of immunosuppressant drugs during and after your operation to reduce the risk of this happening.

As the name suggests, these immunosuppressant drugs suppress or reduce the effectiveness of the immune system (the system that protects the body from attack by viruses, bacteria or other foreign substances). The problem is that, while these drugs help prevent your body from attacking the new heart, they also prevent it from attacking viruses and bacteria, so you'll be more prone to infection. If your body does reject the heart, it is most likely to do so in the first few months after the operation, so you'll be on high doses of anti-rejection drugs at first, which means your risk of infection will be quite high. As the risk of rejection lessens, doctors can usually reduce the dose of some of your medicines, but you'll need to take some immunosuppressants for the rest of your life.

There are many different types of immunosuppressant, all with slightly different actions. Some may cause side effects in some people, and you should report anything unusual to your doctor, who will monitor your medication to make sure the combination and dosage is right for you.

You may also need to take other medicines, such as drugs to lower your cholesterol, usually statins (see Chapter 4), antibiotics and antiviral drugs to reduce the risk of infection, drugs to lower your blood pressure (some immunosuppressants increase blood pressure) and, if you are retaining fluid, a diuretic. As with all medicines, you should check with your doctor or pharmacist before taking any other medication, even herbal or other 'natural' remedies. You also need to read very carefully the patient information leaflets that come with your medicines, as there are some foods or drinks that interact with certain drugs, making them less effective or even causing a toxic effect.

Having a transplanted heart is quite a responsibility, and you'll need to be committed to keeping it as healthy as possible. This means making sure you take all your medicines when you're supposed to, sticking to the advice you're given on diet and exercise, and not missing follow-up appointments. For the first few weeks after the operation, you'll need to stay close to the hospital as you'll need to be seen very frequently. After a while, this will be reduced to a weekly appointment. Your check-ups will become less frequent as time goes on, but you may still need to be seen once or twice a year even some years after your transplant.

Emotional worries

A heart transplant is a major, although relatively straightforward, operation, and it's normal to feel apprehensive or nervous about the procedure. Some people feel more anxious about organ transplants than about other types of major surgery, because of the ethical issues involved. How you feel about receiving a donor heart is something you need to address, and talking through the issues with your family and friends, or perhaps with someone who has already had a transplant, can be extremely helpful.

As we tend to regard the heart as being the emotional centre of ourselves, some people find the idea of having what they regard as 'someone else's heart' as being a bit freaky. The heart is essentially, as we've seen, a lump of muscle; more like a machine, in fact, than anything spiritual or emotional. It cannot change your personality or character. You may feel different after a heart transplant; in particular, you may feel depressed and weepy, but this is likely to be a normal response to major surgery after years of illness – any operation of this size is traumatic, and it's perfectly normal to feel a bit strange afterwards.

Some people are also upset by the idea that, in order for there to be a donor heart available, it means that another person has died. People who have had organ transplants often feel deeply privileged to have been given what they see as a wonderful gift – the gift of life. Some grateful recipients have written to their donor's family and are surprised to learn how comforted the grieving family feels, knowing that their loved one's heart has given another person a new life. Of course, some donor families and recipients prefer not to have any contact, so you should discuss your feelings about this with your transplant team.

41

Pacemakers

If your heart failure is causing or is caused by a heart rhythm disorder; you may benefit from having an artificial pacemaker fitted. Basically, the artificial pacemaker does the same job as the sinoatrial node, the body's natural pacemaker (see Chapter 1). Powered by a lithium battery, the device works by sending electrical impulses through wires connected to the right atrium and to both ventricles to stimulate the heart to contract and to help the four chambers of your heart to beat in time with each other. This is known as resynchronization therapy. Pacemakers either work at a fixed pace, in which case they send out small impulses – called pacing – continuously (this is used in people with no natural pacemaker), or they can work 'on demand', in which case they send an impulse only if they detect a slow or irregular heartbeat, although if the heart's natural pacemaker stops working, they'll pace for as long as needed.

Modern pacemakers only weigh between 25 and 50g and are smaller than a matchbox. Under a local anaesthetic, the wires are inserted through a vein in your shoulder or neck. The cardiologist will guide them into place using an X-ray screen, then connect them to the pacemaker, which is then fitted into a small pouch under the skin, between the skin and the muscle. This is a fairly straightforward procedure but you'll probably need to stay in hospital overnight. After that, you'll need regular check-ups to make sure the pacemaker is working properly.

You mustn't drive for the first week after the procedure and you need to tell the Driver and Vehicle Licensing Agency (DVLA) if you've had a pacemaker fitted. Most people will be able to drive after that as long as there are no other problems or regulations that prevent you from driving. Check with the DVLA.

Pacemakers usually last for 5–10 years, after which you'll need a new one. Most people say they can feel the device, especially at first, and you may find that lying in certain positions is uncomfortable. However, most people get used to their pacemakers quite quickly and, with what will probably be a marked improvement in your symptoms, you should feel much better after the procedure.

Complications

There is a slight risk of developing an infection after a pacemaker is fitted, so you'll probably be given antibiotics immediately before the procedure and for a few days afterwards. If you notice any redness, swelling or discharge at the site where the pacemaker is fitted, it's very important to tell your doctor immediately because a serious infection could mean you have to have the pacemaker removed.

Another possible complication occurs if one of the wires moves out of place and requires repositioning. For this reason, you'll probably be advised to avoid vigorous exercise for a few weeks.

Implantable cardioverter defibrillators

Implantable cardioverter defibrillators (ICDs) work in much the same way as a pacemaker, although the device is larger, weighing about 75g. ICDs tend to be used when the heart beats too quickly or when the chambers of the heart quiver instead of contracting fully. This can be dangerous because when the heart is quivering instead of beating properly, it cannot pump any blood around the body. The defibrillator senses the abnormal rhythm and, if the disturbance is fairly minor, it sends out a short series of small electrical impulses – pacing – to restore a more normal rhythm. If it detects a more serious rhythm disorder, it sends out a stronger impulse to shock the heart into stopping the abnormal beating and resuming a normal rhythm.

The implantation of an ICD is similar to that of a pacemaker, and you should be home within a day or two. Most people are aware of the device inside them and you'll probably feel a fluttering sensation as it delivers pacing impulses. If it has to deliver a larger shock it will probably feel like a heavy thump in the chest. You may find this a little distressing, especially the first time it happens. If you get warning symptoms before the shock is delivered – dizziness or palpitations, for example – you should sit or lie down. After the shock has been delivered and your heart is beating normally again, you may want to rest and recover for a few minutes before getting on with your day.

You must not drive for the first six months after the operation and you must tell the DVLA that you've had a defibrillator fitted. You may be able to resume driving after the first six months as long as there are no other reasons why it might not be safe, although you will have to renew your licence every three years. Check with the DVLA.

You will also need to avoid certain activities that could be dangerous if your ICD were to deliver a shock while you were engaged in them – for example, swimming alone or climbing ladders or scaffolding. If you're unsure, ask your ICD clinic for advice.

Complications

The possible complications after insertion of a defibrillator are similar to those that may be experienced after a pacemaker has been fitted. Rarely, the pulse generator may break through the skin and need to be implanted again. Very occasionally, you may receive one or more inappropriate shocks, sometimes a series of them one after the other. If this happens, you should dial 999 or go to the hospital emergency department.

Left ventricular assist devices

Left ventricular assist devices (LVADs) used to be used only as a temporary treatment for people waiting for a heart transplant, and they were originally quite big, bulky machines. Now, however, smaller versions are available. They are fitted inside the upper abdominal wall and connected to an external power source – a control system that can be worn on a belt and a small battery pack that fits in a shoulder holster.

The left ventricle is responsible for pumping oxygen-rich blood into the aorta, from where it is carried to the heart muscle and to the rest of the body. When the left ventricle fails, the heart muscle and other organs receive an inadequate blood supply. This device works by taking over the job of the left ventricle. It is connected to the ventricle either directly or by a tube. It removes oxygenated blood from the left ventricle and brings the blood to a mechanical pump, which then pumps it into another tube, which is connected to the aorta. Once the oxygen-rich blood is in the aorta, it can be pushed back into the circulatory system to be transported to the rest of the body.

The device is most commonly used in those waiting for a heart transplant, where it is known as a 'bridge to transplantation'. In these cases it is a short-term treatment and is removed after transplantation of a donor heart. In some patients suffering from myocarditis (where a severe virus has weakened the heart muscle) the device may be used to give the heart muscle a 'rest' while it recovers. In these cases, the device will be removed once the heart has fully recovered.

More recently, LVADs are being used as 'artificial hearts' in patients with severe end-stage heart failure who are not suitable for a transplant. In these cases, the device is used for the rest of the patient's life – this is known as 'destination treatment'. At the time of writing, the insertion of this device in patients with end-stage heart failure is a fairly high-risk operation, and it is therefore used only as a last option; it is not suitable for everyone. Only a small number of people in the UK are currently receiving this treatment, although research into its long-term effectiveness is ongoing and in the future it could become a useful treatment in the management of chronic heart failure.

Peter

The first person in the UK to have received an artificial heart for end-stage heart failure is Peter Houghton, now aged 66. Peter underwent the procedure in 2000, and is now in the *Guinness Book of Records* as the longest surviving artificial heart patient:

> I developed heart failure after I had a heart attack when I was 55. I was put on the usual heart drugs, which worked for about three years, but I started to need ever bigger doses. I began to feel tired all the time and generally unwell. I became increasingly breathless even when resting, I could only get around with extreme difficulty and I was swollen up with severe oedema. I was very ill indeed. I'd worked in palliative care, so I recognized the signs, and I knew by this time that I was dying. I'd counselled dying people, so I was prepared – I just hoped it would be quick. Then through a chance meeting with an old colleague, I heard about this new treatment. I was told there was only a 50 per cent chance of success, so I discussed it with my wife and family for about a week, then I decided to go for it. I knew the operation was risky, but by that time, I only had weeks to live anyway.
>
> To be honest, I didn't really expect to survive, so it was quite something to open my eyes after the second day and see my wife

standing there. The first days and weeks were tough; the sedation made me feel like I was in a cocoon, I was wired up to lots of machines and I still felt quite ill. Once or twice I did wonder if I'd done the right thing. But then gradually, over the next few weeks, I became stronger. I learned to walk again and came out of hospital after 11 weeks. A year later, I walked the canal from Birmingham to Oxford to prove that I could!

These days, I can get around much more easily, although there is still an underlying 'unwellness', and of course, having an artificial heart doesn't stop other things going wrong with your body as you get older – I've had kidney and prostate problems recently and I even picked up MRSA a while ago. It's not been an easy six years, but it's six years' more life than I would have had!

Peter has put his extra six years to good use by campaigning to raise money for the Heart Failure Foundation (previously the Artificial Heart Fund) so that more patients might benefit from this treatment, which is very expensive and not yet available on the NHS.

Risks of having heart surgery

All surgical operations carry a certain amount of risk. These risks vary depending on a number of factors, including the type of procedure being carried out, your age and your general state of health. You should discuss the risks and potential benefits of surgery with your surgeon, and with your partner or family before making your decision. In most cases, the risks, if there are any, are small, and doctors recommend a procedure only if they feel that the potential benefits outweigh the risks.

6

How you can help yourself

In addition to the various medications and surgical options to treat heart failure, there are a number of steps that you can take to improve your condition and your general health. Even fairly minor lifestyle changes can make you feel better from day to day and can help prevent your heart failure from getting worse.

Give up smoking

If you've been diagnosed with heart failure, you'll have been told a million times by now and so you'll be sick of hearing it, but let's say it again anyway: give up smoking! Smoking causes the blood vessels to contract, making it even harder for your heart to pump blood around your body. Also, the nicotine and other chemicals in tobacco damage the lining of your arteries so that they are more likely to become 'furred up' with fatty deposits, adding to the narrowing effect. Smoking also raises the blood pressure, making more work for the heart, and it makes the blood stickier and more likely to clot, which not only obstructs the blood vessels yet further, but also increases your risk of a heart attack or stroke.

No one is going to pretend that stopping smoking is easy, especially if you've smoked for a very long time, but it may turn out to be considerably easier than you think. There are several ways to give up smoking, and you should talk to your doctor or heart-care team about which methods are suitable for you. Whichever you choose, you need to make a positive and definite mental commitment to giving up – once you've done that, the battle is half won. In fact, many ex-smokers argue that making the mental decision to quit is the most difficult thing – after that, the rest is surprisingly easy. There is no doubt that nicotine is addictive, and each cigarette you smoke tops up the nicotine levels, making you want even more. But within 48 hours of stopping smoking, almost all the nicotine has left your body, so the 'twitch' you feel after that is no more than a habit. When you think about it, most people go anything between six and eight hours without a cigarette every night – would that be possible if the addiction was the only thing keeping you smoking?

For some people, nicotine replacement therapy (nicotine patches, gum, inhalers, etc) is the answer. This attempts to break the habit first, then allows you to wean yourself off the nicotine slowly. For others, a drug called bupropion (brand name: Zyban) might be the best option. This drug was originally used as an antidepressant, but doctors noticed that many smokers who used it gave up while taking it, and it is now used to help people stop smoking. It's not suitable for everyone, but it may be worth asking your doctor whether it would be likely to help you and whether it would be safe for you to take. Many people give up with the help and support of an anti-smoking group or clinic, or even a telephone support line – studies show that quitters who have support tend to be more successful than those who go it alone. Talk to your doctor about your decision to quit. He or she should be able either to advise you directly or to put you in touch with an anti-smoking clinic or group that will offer professional support and advice. If you prefer a do-it-yourself approach, there are a number of self-help books available (see Further reading, page 111).

A heart-friendly diet

What we eat affects our health in many ways, and bad eating habits can increase the risk of many serious illnesses, including coronary heart disease. As we've already seen, there is very little that can be done to repair damage already done to the heart, but there is a great deal that can be done to prevent heart failure from getting worse and to improve overall health. We're always being told to eat a 'balanced' diet or to 'eat more healthily', but what does this actually mean, and what can you do in practical terms to improve your diet and keep your heart as healthy as possible? There are a number of excellent 'heart health' cookery and recipe books on the market, but even if you're not keen on going into this in a big way, just thinking about food in a different way can help. The following suggestions will help you plan a diet that is healthier for your heart and better for your overall health but that still allows you to enjoy a variety of foods, including the odd treat.

Reduce your salt intake

When you have heart failure, one of the most important changes you can make to your diet is to cut down on the amount of salt that you eat. Too much salt will encourage your body to retain fluid and will work against diuretic medicines (see Chapter 4). A high-salt diet also raises blood pressure, putting an extra strain on the heart.

In the UK, the average adult's daily consumption of salt is around 9g. The government recommends that this should be reduced to a maximum of 6g. If you have heart failure, you may need to reduce your salt intake even more, so talk to your heart failure nurse, doctor or dietitian about this.

Reducing the amount of salt you use is about re-educating your taste buds. If you're used to a large amount of salt in your diet, food with very little salt will taste quite odd for a while, but you will get used to it. It's a bit like people who, having once thought they'd never enjoy a cup of tea without sugar, gave up taking sugar and now find sugared tea undrinkable.

There are two ways of cutting down. If you decide to do it gradually, just slowly reduce the amount of salt you add to food during cooking and at the table until, eventually, you stop adding salt altogether. The other way is more drastic. Although it may seem more difficult at first, doing it in one go might prove easier in the long run. Just give this a try for a couple of weeks and see how you get on: cut out all salty foods such as crisps, salted nuts, stock cubes and processed foods such as soups, pizzas and ready meals; don't use salt at the table; and stop adding it to cooking. It'll be strange at first, and you probably won't enjoy your food as much as usual for a few days, but stick with it. Try using more garlic and other herbs and spices to add flavour. After 2–3 weeks, your taste receptors will be far more sensitive and you'll find foods with too much salt quite unpleasant.

Most of the salt in our diets comes from processed foods rather than salt added at the cooking or serving stage – somewhere between 65 and 85 per cent of our total intake – so in order to keep an eye on how much salt you're eating, you really need to read the labels. But these can be confusing. A recent study found that many people thought that sodium and salt were the same thing. In fact, to find the salt content of a product, you need to multiply the amount of sodium by 2.5. As a rough guide, a food that contains 0.5g of sodium or

1.25g of salt per 100g is considered a high-salt food, whereas 0.1g of sodium or 0.25g of salt per 100g is fine.

Beware, also, of hidden salt – that is, salt found in foods that we don't think of as salty. These include bread, baked beans and some cereals. Other high-salt foods include takeaways, processed meats such as bacon and salami, pork pies, cheese, some pickles and cooking sauces.

Some tips to liven up salt-free food:

- Lemon or lime juice added to olive oil makes a good marinade, especially with added garlic and herbs such as rosemary, thyme, sage or oregano.
- Garlic and other herbs or spices are good rubbed into meat, poultry or fish.
- Olive oil infused with garlic makes a great flavouring for jacket potatoes.
- Try adding a spoonful of tomato puree and some chopped, fresh basil to mashed potatoes, or stir in a spoonful of Dijon mustard.
- Freshly ground black pepper is a great flavouring for many dishes.
- Chilli powder or flakes can be used as a mild flavouring as well as a hot one!

Thinking about cholesterol

We all need a certain amount of fat, but it's the type of fat we eat that has a major bearing on our health, with high cholesterol levels being particularly implicated in heart disease. We need some cholesterol, and the body makes a certain amount itself. The rest comes from the food we eat. After we've eaten a meal, the liver takes cholesterol and triglycerides (the chemical form of some fats) from the blood and packages them into tiny spheres called lipoproteins. The lipoproteins, a combination of cholesterol, trigly-cerides and certain proteins, are transported in the bloodstream to the body cells where the various components are extracted as required.

You'll probably know you should be keeping your cholesterol levels down, but what can confuse the issue is that there are two types of cholesterol, one of which is considered 'bad' cholesterol, which is measured in the blood as low-density lipoprotein (LDL), and one of which is considered 'good' cholesterol, which is measured as high-density lipoprotein (HDL). Most cholesterol in the blood comes from LDL, and when doctors refer to high cholesterol levels, they usually mean LDL. If you have high LDL cholesterol levels, the LDL tends to stick to the lining of the arteries, causing atherosclerosis and a build-up of deposits and leading to narrowed arteries. The 'good' cholesterol comes from HDL, but this usually represents only a small proportion of blood cholesterol. Although we're not certain why HDL is good for you, there is some evidence to suggest that it actually scours the walls of the blood vessels, cleaning out the excess cholesterol and then carrying it back to the liver for further processing.

There are several factors associated with increased levels of LDL cholesterol in your blood, some of which – age, sex and family history – can't be changed. But there are some factors that you can influence, such as giving up smoking (see above), increasing the amount of exercise in your daily routine and changing your diet. Although diet is responsible for only a relatively small amount of cholesterol in the body – most is produced by the liver – a diet that is high in saturated fats can cause the liver to produce more LDL cholesterol. Exactly to what extent diet influences cholesterol levels varies from person to person. In most cases, switching to a low-fat diet will reduce cholesterol levels, but some people on relatively low-fat diets still find it difficult to keep their cholesterol levels under control. Others get away with eating diets outrageously high in fat and still have normal or even low cholesterol levels, which really doesn't seem fair for the rest of us, but that's life.

The worst culprits for increasing LDL cholesterol are saturated fats – those found in animal fats such as meat, lard and dairy products – and it is the intake of saturated fats that heart patients should concentrate on reducing. Unsaturated fats – those that come mainly from plant sources or fish – are much healthier and often contain HDL ('good') cholesterol. Unsaturated fats may be monounsaturated – sources include almonds, hazelnuts and peanut, rapeseed and olive oils – or polyunsaturated, which can be found in soya, sunflower and corn oils, walnuts, seeds, wheat germ and fish oils. Studies show that polyunsaturates and, to a lesser extent, monounsaturates, can help lower blood cholesterol levels.

Some types of fatty acids can't be made within the body but are vital for good health. These are called essential fatty acids –

'essential' because we need to take them in regularly in the form of food. Essential fatty acids are needed for the growth and repair of tissues and for a number of other functions, including skin repair, brain function and immune system functioning.

There are two types of essential fatty acids, omega-3 and omega-6. Good sources of omega-3 fatty acids include soya bean oil and rapeseed oil, as well as fish, especially oily varieties such as sardines, herring, mackerel, trout and salmon. We need around 1–2g per day of omega-3 fatty acids, and this can be provided by a 100g portion of herring or a handful of walnuts. Omega-6 is found in many vegetable oils, especially sunflower, olive oil and corn oil. The daily requirement is about 4g per day, which would be provided by two teaspoons of sunflower oil or a handful of almonds or walnuts.

Essential fatty acids should not be confused with trans fatty acids. Trans fatty acids, like saturated fats, increase cholesterol levels and are therefore detrimental to heart health. Ironically, trans fatty acids are the result of manufacturers trying to make products more healthy. When the dangers associated with saturated fats were identified, the food industry wanted to switch to using unsaturated fatty acids. As unsaturated fatty acids turn rancid so quickly, manufacturers began to hydrogenate them, a process that forms a more solid, longer-lasting form of vegetable oil called partially hydrogenated oil. Unfortunately, a side effect of the process is the formation of another type of fatty acid – trans fatty acid. So when manufacturers began to use partially hydrogenated vegetable oils instead of saturated fats in their processed foods, they began adding large amounts of trans fatty acids. It's fairly easy to identify foods that contain large amounts of trans fatty acids: solid margarines (the harder the margarine, the higher it is in trans fatty acids), high-fat bakery products such as cakes, biscuits and doughnuts, fried foods such as chips and potato crisps, and anything that says 'partially hydrogenated vegetable oil' on the label.

Cut down on fat

Most of us eat too much fat, so try to reduce the total amount of fat in your diet, especially saturated fat. Below are a number of tips to help you to cut down. In addition, read the labels when you're food shopping. As a rough guide, you're fairly safe with foods that have less than 2g of saturated fat per portion. Anything that has 2–5g of saturated fat per portion should be kept as an occasional food, and foods that have more than 5g saturated fat per portion are best avoided altogether if possible. If you're a man, you should be aiming for a maximum of 30g of saturated fat per day (no more than 95g in total fat) and if you're a woman, you need to try and keep to under 20g of saturated fat a day (no more than 70g of total fat). If you're trying to lose weight, you'll probably need to eat less than this. A word of caution – foods that are labelled 'low fat' may be an excellent choice, but do read the label carefully: they may also be high in salt or sugar.

Some tips to help you to cut down on fat:

- Cut down on red meat and choose leaner cuts; trim off visible fat.
- Avoid fatty processed meat products such as sausages and burgers.
- Poultry is a lower fat option – but remove the skin!
- Use skimmed or semi-skimmed milk.
- Use an olive oil-based spread instead of butter or margarine.
- Go easy on the cheese and choose lower-fat cheeses such as edam, brie or half-fat cheddar.
- Poach, grill or bake rather than fry. When stir-frying, use an olive oil spray, or brush the oil on with a pastry brush.
- Choose fat-free salad dressings.
- For desserts, use low fat yoghurt or fromage frais instead of cream or ice cream.
- Have larger portions of vegetables or salad and smaller portions of meat.

Fruit and vegetables

Not only will fruit and vegetables fill you up and provide essential fibre, they are also an excellent source of vitamins, minerals and antioxidants. They'll help to boost your immune system and to protect you against a number of diseases, including several types of cancer. You should eat, at the very least, five portions of fruit and vegetables each day. One serving of fruit is one item such as an apple or an orange, or a handful of berries, or a small glass of fruit juice. One large carrot or a medium portion of salad or greens counts as one serving of vegetables.

The best possible way to eat these healthy foods is raw or lightly cooked and with no dressing. Avoid vegetables that have been cooked in saturated fat, vegetables served with butter, and salads with oily or creamy dressings. For stir-fries or roasting, use a small amount of olive, sunflower or rapeseed oil. Dress salads with a tiny amount of olive oil and lemon juice, or use fat-free dressings.

Try for a couple of pieces of fruit a day and at least three portions of vegetables. If you're one of those people who refers to anything green or crunchy as 'rabbit food', think about sneaky ways of increasing your intake. Try making vegetable soups. They're very easy to make – often simply a combination of two or three vegetables and some stock and seasoning. Simmer the chopped vegetables in the stock until soft, then whisk in a blender for a smooth soup or leave chunky if you prefer. Or you can find simple recipes in books, in magazines, in the supermarket or on the internet. Try these simple but delicious soup ideas: carrot and coriander, curried parsnip or butternut squash, broccoli or butternut squash and soft cheese with garlic and herbs (low-fat version), roasted red pepper and garlic, leek and potato, French onion, or tomato and carrot. Try adding extra vegetables to casseroles, stews, curries and pasta sauces. Chargrilled Mediterranean vegetables go well with fish or on a thin-crust pizza, or you could throw a handful of mushrooms or sweet corn into an omelette, pile coleslaw into a jacket potato, or have baked beans or tomatoes on toast for breakfast. If you think salads are boring, have a look on the internet or get a good recipe book from the library and try experimenting with some more unusual salad combinations, but don't forget you'll need to stick to low-fat or fat-free dressings.

To boost your fruit intake, start each day with a glass of fruit juice and add some chopped fruit to your cereal or yoghurt in the mornings. For desserts, try adding chopped fruit to fromage frais or low-fat ice-cream, or you could make a big fresh fruit salad. Don't forget that dried fruit such as prunes or apricots counts towards your daily intake.

Starchy carbohydrates

Starchy carbohydrates, such as bread, cereal, rice, pasta and potatoes, provide the most energy. Depending on your height and weight, you should eat between six and 11 servings from this group each day. One slice of bread or a small bowl of cereal counts as a serving.

The biggest danger with this food group is that it's the one to which we are most likely to add fat without really noticing, so you need to keep an eye on how you cook and serve your carbohydrates and what you're eating with them. Avoid deep fried or thinly cut chips, potatoes cooked in cream, small potatoes roasted in saturated fat, pasta served with butter or cream-based sauces, and fried rice. Occasional small portions of reduced-fat oven chips or of potatoes roasted in a tiny amount of olive oil are probably all right, and although tomato-based sauces are the best option with pasta, you can probably get away with a cheesy sauce now and again, as long as you stick to small portions and don't have it too often.

Milk and dairy foods

Milk and other dairy foods are good providers of calcium for healthy bones and of some protein, but they can also be very high in fat. Have two or three portions a day, and choose the lower fat options where possible – for example skimmed or semi-skimmed milk, low-fat or fat-free yoghurt, half-fat cheddar, half-fat edam, cottage cheese, ricotta cheese, or 'light' or 'extra light' soft cheese. A small pot of yoghurt, a medium glass of milk or a matchbox-sized piece of medium fat cheese counts as a portion. Some soft cheeses such as brie or camembert should be all right for an occasional treat, but check that they have less than 30g total fat per 100g. When you have heart problems, you really do need to steer clear of cream – clotted, double, whipped and even single, pouring cream. Watch out for cream substitutes with a high fat content. As a special treat, have the odd full-fat yoghurt or fromage frais, or allow yourself a little half-fat cream – but don't treat yourself too often.

Meat and poultry

These foods should form a smaller part of your meal, which should be bulked up with lots of vegetables or salad, plus some carbohydrate such as rice, pasta or potatoes. Choose lean cuts of meat and serve it grilled, dry-roasted, stir-fried or in a casserole. Aim for one or two portions a day, and try to only eat meat on 2–3 days a week, choosing fish or non-meat alternatives on other days. A portion of meat is a piece about the size of a pack of playing cards. Remove the skin from chicken and turkey, and try to avoid the fattier birds such as duck and goose. Corned beef is probably best avoided, as are sausages and burgers, although if you really can't live without them, low-fat or 'healthy-eating' versions can be an occasional treat.

Fish

Fish is good! Unless, of course, it's swimming in a butter- or cream-based sauce, or it's been battered or bread-crumbed and deep-fried. Frozen fish in 'oven-bake' batter or breadcrumbs is okay now and again, but go easy as these varieties can be high in fat and salt. You should also limit the amount of shellfish you eat because, although shellfish is low in fat, the small amount that is present is in the form of cholesterol and may affect your cholesterol levels. Opt for grilled, steamed, baked or poached fish, and try to have one portion of white fish and one portion of oily fish (such as salmon, trout, mackerel or sardines) each week. Tinned fish (drained of oil) is also a good option.

Eggs

Eggs are fairly high in cholesterol, but that doesn't mean you can't have them at all. Most experts agree that three or four eggs a week are fine. Boiled, poached or scrambled with a small amount of milk and low-fat spread (not butter!) are the best choice. The occasional fried egg won't hurt you, as long as you fry it in a small amount of rapeseed, olive or sunflower oil.

Nuts

If you like to eat nuts as an alternative to meat, opt for walnuts, chestnuts, almonds or hazelnuts. Keep pistachios, pecans and peanuts, and peanut butter, for an occasional treat, and try to avoid the really high-fat nuts such as Brazil nuts, cashews and coconut (including coconut milk).

Beans, peas and lentils

Beans, peas and lentils are excellent sources of protein and fibre. Tinned or dried kidney beans, haricot beans, black eye beans, chick peas and lentils are all good choices, including tinned baked beans in tomato sauce. Vegetarian burgers and bean-burgers are okay now and again, but they can have a fairly high fat content. Exercise caution when eating out – Indian dahls and chick pea curries in particular can be very high in fat and are often made with large amounts of ghee (clarified butter).

Sweets, desserts, cakes and biscuits

This is the food group from which we should eat the most sparingly. We all like a little something sweet now and again, but some of these little treats are absolutely oozing fat, even if they sound quite healthy. Flapjacks, for example, often contain a lot of butter or margarine. For teatime snacks, it's best to stick to the plainer biscuits, such as rich tea or malted milk, plain fat-free sponge cake or dried fruits. If you must have a dessert, opt for jelly, baked apples, or fresh or stewed fruit. If you want to feel as if you're having a naughty dessert, try piling fresh strawberries or raspberries onto a meringue nest and topping with a little low-fat fromage frais.

Although there is no direct link between sugar and heart disease, sugar is a high-calorie food with virtually no nutritional value. In large quantities it can make you gain weight – not good for someone with a heart problem – and rot your teeth. It really is best all round to keep sugary foods to a minimum.

Drink alcohol in moderation

Unless the damage to your heart was actually caused by drinking too much alcohol (in which case your doctor will advise you to abstain completely from now on), drinking a small amount of alcohol shouldn't do you any harm. However, alcohol can worsen some heart failure symptoms – for example, dizziness and fatigue. The key is *moderate* consumption – in other words, no more than two units a day for women, three for men. If you're watching your weight, you may need to have less alcohol than this, because alcohol is fairly high in calories and, like sugar, it has little nutritional value. You should also have at least two alcohol-free days a week. There is much speculation on whether the type of alcohol you drink has any bearing on how good or bad it is for the heart. There is some evidence to suggest that red wine may prevent the blood from becoming sticky and may increase the levels of HDL ('good') cholesterol, although more research is needed on this subject. If you have a problem with swelling, watch the amount of fluid you drink, especially if you like to drink beer. Alcohol may also affect your medication – it increases the effects of warfarin, for example – so do talk to your doctor or heart-care team about what a safe level of alcohol consumption would be. One unit of alcohol is roughly half a pint of normal-strength beer or lager, a small glass (125ml) of wine, a pub measure (25ml) of spirits or half a glass (50ml) of fortified wine such as port or sherry.

Watch your weight

When you have heart failure, you need to keep a very close eye on your weight, because a sudden increase – more than 2kg in a couple of days – could be an indication that your body is retaining fluid. Weigh yourself each morning after you've emptied your bladder and, if you notice a sudden change or if you notice increased breathlessness or swelling in your feet and ankles, tell your doctor or heart failure nurse so that the cause can be established as quickly as possible. If you have a tendency to retain fluid, you will be advised to limit the amount you have to drink each day, at least until the situation is under control.

Keep active

In the past, it was often thought that exercise was dangerous for people with heart failure, and therefore patients were advised to take lots of rest and avoid exerting themselves. Now, we know that regular, moderate exercise is actually helpful. In fact, many cardiac rehabilitation programmes now include exercise sessions. If you don't attend one of these programmes, you should talk to your doctor or heart failure nurse about the amount of exercise you should do and whether there's anything you should avoid, especially if you have other health problems or are seriously overweight.

Research on the benefits of exercise for people with heart failure shows that exercise can actually strengthen your heart and improve its pumping ability, thus increasing the amount of blood flowing through your heart and the amount of oxygen going around your body. Muscles need oxygen to keep fit, and exercise will improve muscle fitness and build up muscle strength so that you can move around more without getting tired. Exercise also tends to lower blood pressure and helps to keep your joints flexible.

As well as helping you to feel physically fitter, exercise also has a beneficial effect on the mind, helping to combat depression by causing the brain to release certain 'happy chemicals' – hormones that lift mood – into the bloodstream. It also helps to reduce stress, improve memory and boost confidence.

We're not talking about signing up for the gym here or starting your own football or hockey team, just about finding ways of gradually increasing your fitness and stamina from where you are at the moment. Even getting out of the chair and walking around the living room a couple of times can improve your fitness if you've been immobile for a long time. Unless you've been told by your doctor to rest completely, any extra movement will help.

Little and often

It's very important to build up your fitness gradually in order to avoid the 'overactivity–rest cycle'. This happens when you overdo things because you're feeling well, then you have to rest for the next day or two because you overdid it on the first day. Supposing, for example, you wake up one sunny Sunday morning feeling better than you have in weeks; you head out into the garden intending to do a bit of light weeding and pruning, but you feel so good that you dig over two flower beds, cut the hedge, mow the lawn and even seriously consider cleaning out the pond. It's natural to want to get as much done as possible when you're feeling energetic, especially if you don't have the energy very often. But if you do this, whatever fitness you gained by doing the gardening will soon be lost as you have to reduce your activity levels over the next few days in order to recover. Fitness is lost far more quickly than it is gained, so even if you're only out of action for a day or two, you'll find it harder to get started again than you would if you'd only done 10 minutes of activity every day.

The best way to avoid this is to work out an amount that you can do easily every day and then build up gradually from there. Much will depend on how fit you are when you start. If, for example, you decide that a 20-minute walk would be a good starting point but you find that you can only walk for 15 minutes without becoming breathless, then lower your starting point to 15 minutes. After a few days, increase that to 17 or 18 minutes, then to 20, then to 25 and so on. If you do this every day, your fitness will increase slowly but consistently, and you should notice a significant difference in a few weeks. If you take a break for some reason, you'll need to return to a low starting point: if you've been walking for an hour a day, then you become ill and can't go out for a couple of weeks, your fitness levels will fall; don't try to pick up where you left off, simply go back to your original 15-minute starting point and slowly build up again. If you suddenly feel ill or unreasonably tired, or if your symptoms are getting worse, tell your doctor straight away.

It can be quite difficult to stop yourself from overdoing it when you're feeling well, but you really must be strict with yourself. Plan the amount of activity you're going to take and don't do any more, even if you feel fine. The following day, you can increase the amount you do by a little, and if you're comfortable with that amount after a few days, increase a little more and so on.

When deciding what activities are best, you need to take into account your level of heart failure, your current fitness and the sort of things you enjoy doing. If you're fairly fit, something like swimming or dancing might be the thing. If those types of activity are too strenuous, perhaps gentle walking or a yoga class might be more appropriate. Choose something that you know you can keep up rather than something you'll only do for a short time – the most important thing is to exercise regularly, even if it's only for a few minutes every day. Think about the sort of person you are and the things you enjoy doing. Do you like the great outdoors or are you more of an indoor person? Are you sociable and outgoing or are you happier in your own company or that of a partner or close friend? What about your children or grandchildren? Could you combine spending quality time with the children with an activity that would help you to get fit? Thinking about your work, hobbies, interests, family and friends may give you some ideas as to how to devise the most appropriate way to include exercise in your daily routine. As your fitness increases, you may find that you can progress to other activities. In the mean time, think about your existing routine. Do you go out to work or is your day's activity centred around the home? Could you walk part of the way to work or to the shops? Park the car a little further away? Get off the bus or train one stop earlier? If you took just a 15-minute walk every day – perhaps a $7\frac{1}{2}$-minute walk each way to the newsagent for a paper – you'll have clocked up almost 2 hours of exercise at the end of the week.

Exercise tips

Here are some tips for exercising:

- Check with your doctor or heart failure nurse before embarking on a new exercise programme.
- Any exercise is worth doing. If you can only manage to walk to the end of the garden and back, go for it. No matter how small the amount of exercise, you can rejoice in the fact that you are building up your fitness and improving the efficiency of your heart.
- Be realistic about what you can achieve, and start each activity at the level that's right for you.
- Exercise regularly, increasing your activity slowly. Plan your exercise sessions and do no more than you'd planned, even if you feel like it.
- If you're not well, go back to a lower level of activity until you feel better, then build up again gradually.
- Don't do anything too vigorous such as squash or weightlifting – sudden, hard physical effort can raise your blood pressure.
- Stop if you feel pain or any more than slight breathlessness. It's normal to become a little breathless while exercising, but you should stop if you feel uncomfortably breathless. You should also stop if you feel faint or if you experience any chest pain. If you are in any doubt at all about whether it is safe to continue, talk to your doctor.
- Always warm up first and cool down after exercise so that you don't damage ligaments or muscles. Start with gentle stretches or by walking slowly for the first few minutes, then slow down again at the end of the session.
- Don't exercise for an hour or so after eating.
- If in doubt, ask your health-care team for advice.

While it's important to exercise every day it's equally important to vary the type of exercise you do to avoid boredom setting in. Here are some activity ideas for you to think about:

- Walking – a very flexible form of exercise that you can do alone, with your partner, your children or grandchildren, a walkers' group or just the dog. You don't need any special skill or expertise and you can start very gradually by walking around the house or garden a little more. You'll soon notice you're able to go further. As you become fitter, you might want to invest in a pedometer, an inexpensive device that clips on to your belt or waistband and measures the number of steps you take. It's a great motivational tool and will encourage you to go, if not the 'extra mile', at least an extra few steps.

- Take up golf – it may seem a gentle occupation, but the average golf course is 3–4 miles long, so walking around it can be quite a workout! If you've never played before, it would be worth taking a few lessons. Injuries are rare, but strains and sprains do sometimes occur in golfers who haven't learned how to move their bodies properly while perfecting their swing.
- Swimming – particularly good if you're overweight or have back problems. Swimming is an excellent non-weight-bearing exercise. The water supports you making injury less likely, and you can build up from a width or two of the pool to several lengths.
- Cycling – another great non-weight-bearing exercise and a cheap form of transport as well.
- Tai chi – based on ancient Chinese healing and martial arts, tai chi involves gentle, controlled movements and is a form of exercise particularly well suited to people who find more strenuous exercise difficult. In tai chi, weight is transferred slowly from one flexed leg to the other, helping blood to return to the heart as well as improving muscle strength and control.

In fact, several studies have been carried out on the use of tai chi to treat people with heart failure, and early indications are encouraging. A recent US study found that heart failure patients who attended tai chi classes twice a week for 12 months had improved mobility and reduced levels of natriuretic peptide. In a statement issued in early 2006, Belinda Linden, head of medical information at the British Heart Foundation, said:

There have been some very positive results from studies on tai chi programmes, particularly in their role in encouraging physical activity in patients with heart conditions. The benefits from tai chi may not only include the impact of physical activity on heart health, but also the positive social support that comes from a group activity and the commitment involved. Large studies are in progress in the US and the UK to assess the benefits of tai chi for specific groups of patients such as those with heart failure. There are immense benefits in getting more active, however, all activity needs to be introduced and increased gradually so that it can be tailored to each person's ability.

And if you're not ready to embark on any of these forms of exercise yet, think about other ways to increase your activity levels. Even if you have seriously reduced mobility because of age, weight or illness, you can still perform some stretching or muscle-strengthening exercises while sitting in a chair, perhaps to music to make it more interesting. Talk to your doctor or heart failure nurse about devising a suitable set of movements.

Avoiding infection

When you have heart failure, you need to be extra careful to avoid infections such as flu, bronchitis or other chest infections. You should consider getting a flu jab before each winter, and also immunization against pneumococcus – a bacterium that is one of the causes of pneumonia. Talk to your doctor or the practice nurse about when you should do this. If you've had an operation on your heart, you may need to take antibiotics before you have other surgery of any kind, including dental surgery, to avoid the risk of infection.

Keep taking the tablets

It's very important to keep taking your various medications when you have heart failure, even if you feel much better. It's also important to stay in touch with your health-care team so that they can monitor your condition and make any changes necessary in your treatment. One of the main reasons that people who are already being treated for heart failure end up in hospital is because they stop taking their tablets or don't take them correctly. Remember:

- Take your medicines as directed, whether you feel well or unwell.
- Don't stop taking any of your medicines unless your doctor or heart failure nurse tells you to.
- Remind your doctor which medicines you are taking.
- Tell your doctor or heart failure nurse if you develop any side effects from your medicines – don't just stop taking them.
- If you take any other medicine or remedy, including herbal remedies and over-the-counter preparations for colds, pain or heartburn, always check with your doctor or heart failure nurse.

Heart failure is an ongoing illness, so although once your condition is stable you'll be able to relax a little, you'll still need to be quite vigilant about your treatment, general health and lifestyle.

7

Reaction to diagnosis

Being diagnosed with heart failure can be a nasty shock, even if you're already aware that you have heart problems. If, for example, you've already had a heart attack, you will have been concentrating on recovery, perhaps planning a whole new way of life to protect your heart in the future. To then be told that your heart has been damaged beyond repair is understandably depressing. Even though, as we've seen throughout this book, a diagnosis of heart failure doesn't mean you'll never be able to enjoy life again, it is something you'll need time to come to terms with.

John
When John, aged 45, was diagnosed with heart failure a year ago, after almost two years of tests and investigations, he wasn't sure how he felt at first:

I know it sounds crazy, but my first reaction to the diagnosis was relief. I'd been so ill for a long time, and I'd been tested for everything from anaemia to black water fever! I'd felt generally tired and unwell for ages, and had so little energy that I could barely get up a flight of stairs without feeling like I'd run a marathon.

I was at the hospital for yet another round of tests when my doctor came in and said, 'John, we have good news and bad news.' At the time, I thought the bad news would be that I had cancer – I don't know what I thought the good news would be! I was so pleased that it wasn't cancer and so relieved that they finally knew what was wrong, I didn't really take it in at first. Of course, over the next few weeks, it sunk in.

In my case, the heart failure is quite severe, so I've had to come to terms with the fact that I may not live to a ripe old age, although my doctor says some people with serious heart failure do survive for quite some time. Maybe things would have been better if it had been diagnosed earlier, but it may not have made any difference. I don't blame the doctors for not spotting it sooner – given that I've never had a heart attack or any other heart problem, I'm very young to have heart failure. Also, I'd always been very healthy, I'm not overweight, I've never smoked and apart from a couple of beers at the weekend, I don't really drink, so there was no real reason for them to look for a heart problem. They're baffled as to why I've got it, but they think it may have been caused by a virus. The point is, the reason is not important; I have it, and that's that. I went through a few weeks of being angry, and a few months of being depressed. But I'm beginning to get to grips with the diagnosis now. I concentrate on eating healthily, walking the dog every day to keep myself active and trying out new hobbies – I've taken up painting, which I absolutely love. The hardest thing has been having to give up work and live on benefits, especially when people who don't know see me out and about during the daytime – I'm sure some of them think I'm skiving. Also, it's difficult for my wife Tina, not only is she worried about me, but she's also having to take on a lot of the little jobs and chores I'd have dealt with in the past.

Accepting that I have severe heart failure hadn't been easy, but on the positive side, I now take each day as it comes, and I enjoy every minute of my life.

John's experience of feeling angry and then feeling depressed is a fairly typical one. It's also quite normal to wonder if the doctors have made a mistake. Unfortunately, they almost certainly haven't, so the best thing you can do is to accept that you have heart failure and start thinking about how you can prevent it from getting worse and how you can improve your general health and quality of life. This book ought to help with these things.

Another common reaction is guilt. You may think that if only you'd stopped smoking sooner, if only you'd given up your stressful job, lost that extra weight, not eaten so many burgers . . .

Basically, we can all find a dozen reasons to blame ourselves when things go wrong. It may be true that you wouldn't have heart failure if you'd given up smoking, but it may also be true that it would have made no difference whatsoever. Hitting yourself over the head with notions of what you should have done really won't do anybody any good at all, so give yourself a break!

Facing up to severe illness

If your heart failure is very severe and difficult to treat, you may be faced with the prospect of a limited lifespan. Nobody wants to hear that they're unlikely to live for much longer, but if that is what you've been told, it may help to address your fears by thinking and talking about your situation.

Death is something we must all face, and yet most of us tend not to talk about it, much less prepare for it. The shock of having to confront your own death can be enormous, especially if you are relatively young, maybe even with a family and dependants. You are likely to experience a turmoil of emotions, including those that you experienced when you were first diagnosed with heart failure, only about ten times stronger. You may, of course, have had some idea that your outlook was poor, but even so, being told this officially can be a significant shock.

Many people have a natural fear of death, based largely on the fact that it is the great unknown, and the unknown can be frightening. In addition, you may have fears about your symptoms becoming worse and about what will happen to your partner and family after you die. The best way to deal with these fears is to bring them out into the open and talk about them, thus making them less 'unknown'.

Discuss your medical treatment with your health-care team or the palliative care team if there is one in your area. Palliative care is for people whose illness cannot be cured; it focuses on controlling symptoms and offering emotional support to patients and their families and on providing support in hospital, at home, in a hospice or palliative support unit. You may want to talk about what is likely to happen towards the end and what can be done to alleviate any unpleasant symptoms, as well as where you would prefer to be cared for.

Talking to your loved ones is very important at this time. You, and they, are bound to feel sad; there will probably be tears on more than one occasion, but you will all draw comfort from sharing your feelings with one another. You may also find that talking to a member of the clergy or another spiritual figure is both comforting and supportive, even if you are not affiliated with any particular religion.

If you are worried about the future and how your partner will cope after your death, you may find it helpful to deal with some of the issues now. Making a will is a sensible idea and can be done simply and fairly cheaply. It can be a relief to know that your wishes will be known and your finances dealt with. Some people like to plan their own funeral, while others would prefer to leave the choices to their loved ones. You don't have to make these decisions immediately, but they are things you may want to think about and talk through with your partner and family.

If you have access to the internet, there is a website called 'If I should die' at http://www.ifishoulddie.co.uk, which you may find useful (see page 107). This website has been set up mainly to help bereaved relatives, but it contains a great deal of practical information and advice on death and bereavement, as well as a section offering 'poems and words of comfort'.

Many people in our culture find death and dying difficult to discuss, which is sad, given that it is one thing that every one of us will experience. In cultures where the subject is not taboo, many people face death without fear, seeing it as simply moving on to another stage of being. Whether you agree with this or not, the idea may be of some comfort to you and to your loved ones.

Depression and anxiety

If you are diagnosed with heart failure, you're more likely to suffer from depression, anxiety and mood swings than someone who doesn't have the condition. It is possible that people who develop depression already have a tendency to the illness even before they're diagnosed with heart failure. But what is known for certain is that depression can occur as a result of trauma and distress, and a diagnosis of heart failure can indeed be traumatic and distressing. You're more at risk of depression if you live alone, if you have a history of alcohol misuse, if your heart failure is severe or if you are experiencing financial hardship (see page 79) as a result of your condition.

It's important to recognize that depression is a serious, potentially life-threatening illness in itself, and if you have heart failure as well, depression can affect the way you manage your condition. For example, if you have depression, you're less likely to take physical exercise, you may forget or not bother to take your medication and you're more likely to smoke, drink too much alcohol or eat unhealthily ('comfort eating'). This can lead to a worsening of your heart failure.

The term 'depression' is an overused and often misused one, resulting in a widespread misunderstanding of the illness and a failure to take it seriously. This may explain the stigma that seems to attach to it in the UK, and the resultant reluctance on the part of sufferers to seek help for their depression. There is a huge difference between being depressed and simply feeling 'a bit down'. It's often easier to recognize the signs in someone else than in yourself, so if you think you may be at risk – if you've suffered from it in the past, for example – talk to your family and friends about it. That way, they can be alert to any signs and symptoms that you might miss.

How to recognize depression

We all feel low sometimes, and knowing that you have heart failure can lead to feelings of sadness, of loss of control and of lost youth, as well as fears about any forthcoming heart surgery and the knowledge that you may have to drastically change your lifestyle. You may have been feeling unwell for months, you may be experiencing reduced capacity in your daily life, feeling like you're forever at the doctor's or at hospital, or you may be adjusting to a number of different medications. Each of these things is unsettling. You may feel quite miserable about it all and you have every right to be. But in normal circumstances, you'd gradually start to feel less sad as you discovered more about your illness and treatment, and eventually you would go back to having the odd 'off' day, like most people.

However, if you continue to feel very sad, bleak or hopeless for longer than a few days, you may have depression. The manifestation of the illness varies from person to person, but these are some of the signs to look out for:

- Persistent low mood, often worse in the mornings
- Tearfulness
- Feeling unable to experience pleasure or enjoyment
- Loss of interest in social and work activities
- Reduced or increased appetite

- Sleep difficulties – sleeplessness or early morning wakening, or markedly increased need for sleep
- Lack of energy, fatigue
- Slowed thinking, speech or movements
- Inability to concentrate
- Anxiety or panic attacks
- Feelings of worthlessness and hopelessness
- Being able to only see the negative side of things
- Suicidal thoughts

You don't need to experience all of these symptoms to be suffering from depression, and indeed some of them – lack of energy and fatigue, for example – may be more to do with your heart failure than with depression. However, if you think it may be depression, talk to your doctor about treatment. If you have depression, the chemicals in your brain that govern your mood make it impossible for you simply to 'cheer up'. In fact, telling someone with depression to cheer up or pull himself or herself together is like telling someone with a broken leg to go for a run.

Depression is a serious illness that requires treatment, possibly with medication, counselling or cognitive behaviour therapy, or with a combination of these therapies. Self-help books may also be useful – in fact a 'books-on-prescription' scheme launched in Devon in 2004 had such encouraging results that the scheme is now being used in other areas across the UK. Your doctor will be able to tell you if the scheme operates in your area; if it does, the books should be available at your local library.

The most important thing to remember is that, while depression may be a normal reaction to a diagnosis of heart failure, this does not mean it will go away by itself, although it does in some cases. The good news is that it can be successfully treated in the majority of cases. It may take several months or even a year or more, and if you're treated with antidepressants, it's important to continue taking them for at least six months after you last had symptoms, and then to reduce the dose gradually rather than just stopping. If your doctor prescribes antidepressants, remind him or her of what heart medication you're taking.

Getting help for your depression should improve things for you and your family: not only will you feel better and be able to enjoy life once more, you'll also be better able to manage your heart failure, thus reducing the risk of hospitalization.

Note that there are some herbal preparations that are recommended for mild to moderate depression, and you should not take these without checking with your doctor. St John's wort, for example, while being an effective and gentle treatment for depression, may affect the action of some of your heart failure drugs.

8

Coping on a daily basis

The extent to which your heart failure affects your daily life will depend on the severity of your condition. Some people with fairly mild heart failure find that it barely affects their life at all, while others may find they are unable to work or to enjoy their usual activities. This can be difficult on a number of levels. Clearly, if you need a lot of time off work or you have to give up your job altogether because of your heart failure, this will have an impact on your finances and, possibly, on your sense of self-worth. Similarly, if you have already retired, there may be things that you have always done around the home – shopping, cooking, mowing the lawn, redecorating – that you cannot do any more.

Accepting that your condition puts limitations on your physical activities can be very difficult, but things may not be as bad as they seem. You may find that you can still carry on the same activities but that you have to do smaller amounts and take lots of breaks. If symptoms such as pain and breathlessness become troublesome, for example, it may be that your treatment can be adjusted to alleviate this. The most important thing to remember is to keep in touch with your health-care team, so the difficulties that you experience can be relieved wherever possible.

Stress

Stress sometimes occurs when we feel out of control of a situation and unable to cope with the demands placed on us. This can occur as a result of problems at work, major events such as divorce, bereavement or moving house, difficulties in family relationships, financial problems and your own or your partner's illness (to name but a few). Being diagnosed with heart failure can in itself be stressful, as can coping with the symptoms, so it is important to be aware of this possibility and to have a plan for managing stressful events and situations.

8

Coping on a daily basis

The extent to which your heart failure affects your daily life will depend on the severity of your condition. Some people with fairly mild heart failure find that it barely affects their life at all, while others may find they are unable to work or to enjoy their usual activities. This can be difficult on a number of levels. Clearly, if you need a lot of time off work or you have to give up your job altogether because of your heart failure, this will have an impact on your finances and, possibly, on your sense of self-worth. Similarly, if you have already retired, there may be things that you have always done around the home – shopping, cooking, mowing the lawn, redecorating – that you cannot do any more.

Accepting that your condition puts limitations on your physical activities can be very difficult, but things may not be as bad as they seem. You may find that you can still carry out the same activities, but that you have to do smaller amounts and take lots of breaks. If symptoms such as pain and breathlessness become troublesome, for example, it may be that your treatment can be adjusted to alleviate this. The most important thing to remember is to keep in touch with your health-care team so the difficulties that you experience can be relieved wherever possible.

Stress

Stress sometimes occurs when we feel out of control of a situation and unable to cope with the demands placed on us. This can occur as a result of problems at work; major events such as divorce, bereavement or moving house; difficulties in family relationships; financial problems; and your own or your partner's illness (to name but a few). Being diagnosed with heart failure can in itself be stressful, as can coping with the symptoms, so it's important to be aware of this possibility and to have a plan for managing stressful events and situations.

How stress affects the heart

Stress causes the release of certain hormones that can raise blood pressure, thus increasing the risk of blood clotting in the arteries. Like depression, stress can also make you more likely to smoke, drink too much alcohol and eat unhealthily – all of which are, as we have seen, bad for your heart.

How to recognize stress

Everyone experiences stress differently, and not all stress is bad. For example, changing jobs or even going on holiday can be stressful, but these are also situations that we can find enjoyable. The problem is that, if you're also experiencing 'bad' stress – relationship difficulties, illness, financial problems and so on – even the so-called good stress can be hard to handle. It's important to learn to recognize the symptoms and to act to reduce the harmful stress as soon as possible.

Stress affects different people in different ways, but some common symptoms are:

- Feeling sweaty or shivery
- Panic attacks
- Nausea or 'butterflies' in the stomach
- Palpitations
- Dry mouth
- Headaches
- Unexplained aches and pains
- Extreme tiredness and lack of energy
- Loss of appetite – for food, sex or fun
- Loss of sense of interest in friends, hobbies or appearance
- Irritability
- Forgetfulness or an inability to concentrate
- Sleep disturbances
- Tearfulness
- Hopelessness
- Feeling unable to cope

If you're experiencing five or more of these symptoms, you may be suffering from stress and should take action now. You'll notice that some of these symptoms are similar to those of depression, and

74

indeed the two conditions are often closely linked, although they are not the same thing. Stress can be a major cause of depression, although not everyone who is stressed will suffer from depression, and not everyone with depression will have experienced stress.

If you think your depression is caused by stress, dealing with that stress may help, but you may still need extra help to deal with your depression, so do talk to your doctor about this.

What can you do about stress?

Firstly, you need to identify the possible causes, such as:

- Relationships – difficulties in relationships with your partner, children, friends, colleagues or even neighbours can take their toll.
- Work – having a heavy workload, feeling undervalued and workplace bullying can all be causes of stress at work. Also, work may be the place where the symptoms of stress become noticeable, and can result in poor performance, lack of concentration or taking lots of sick leave (or wanting to, at least).
- Health – whether it's your own heart failure, another health issue or ill health in someone you're close to, this can be a major factor in feeling stressed.
- Financial difficulties – even though most medical treatment in the UK is free, ill health can put a heavy strain on your finances, resulting in a rapid build-up of debt, which can cause severe stress.
- Major life-events – such as changing jobs, retirement, moving house, divorce, children leaving home or bereavement – can all be stressful on their own, but when two or more happen at once, it can really be too much.

Obviously there are some things that can't be changed, but once you've identified the possible cause of your stress, try to find ways of improving the situation. For example, if your workload is too heavy, can you delegate? Can you discuss the situation with your boss? Are there issues at work that could be tackled by your union? If you're worried about debt, could you get financial advice from an organization such as your local Citizens Advice Bureau or the National Debtline (see page 108).

If there's nothing you can do to reduce the source of your stress, there are steps you can take to help you cope with it.

Look after your body

Take a little gentle exercise each day (with guidance from your health-care team), eat as healthily as possible and cut down on alcohol. Give up smoking if you haven't already done so – you may think a cigarette relieves stress, but the effect is temporary and smoking actually increases the symptoms of stress!

Rest and relaxation

None of us is very good at resting and relaxing, but it's essential to allow your body and mind to recharge and recover when you're experiencing stress. If you have a heavy workload, you may say that you don't have time to relax, but several studies have shown that people who take breaks and know how to 'switch off' are able to achieve as much as, and often more than, those people who never stop. If it's practicable, joining a yoga, meditation or relaxation class may help. Book a relaxing massage if funds allow or, if you don't fancy that, at least factor in some time every day for a relaxing activity that you enjoy. The activity might be seeing friends, reading or just listening to music, but make sure it's time spent unwinding – in other words, listening to music while you're doing the ironing doesn't count!

Time management and stress management courses

If you constantly find that there aren't enough hours in the day, or if you feel as if you're trying to run up the down escalator all the time, you may need some professional help in managing your time. There are a number of books on the market that may help, and there are also classes available. Stress management classes may be an even better idea. These may include time management, relaxation techniques and assertiveness training – with valuable advice on how to say 'no'. Classes may also help you to learn how to handle different types of stress and how to manage attitudes and behaviours that create or increase stress. For details of courses near you, contact the International Stress Management Association (see page 107).

Support

When you're coping with stress, you need support; simply talking through the problems with your partner, a friend or another family member can help. Some people are better at listening than others, just as there are some people whose advice you can trust and others whose words of wisdom you have learned to take with a pinch of salt (figuratively speaking, of course – salt is bad for your heart!).

In some situations, a professional counsellor may be the best person to talk to, especially if you're having problems with personal relationships. Another good option might be a support group where you can talk to people who are going through a similar experience. There are support groups for all sorts of life events such as divorce and bereavement, as well as for thousands of different medical conditions, including heart failure. For details of your nearest 'heart support group', contact the British Heart Foundation (see page 106). Many of these groups also welcome partners and close family members.

Having to give up work

If your heart failure is severe or your symptoms become worse as a result of your job, your doctor may advise you (or order you!) to give up your job permanently. It may be that the type of job you do has an adverse effect on your health – if the work is too strenuous, for example. If this is the case, maybe there are other forms of paid work that you could do without risking your health, possibly on a part-time basis. Talk to your doctor or heart failure nurse about this so that you know what your options are.

If you do have to give up work completely, there will obviously be a number of implications for you and your family, including boredom, feelings of inadequacy, relationship problems (see Chapter 9), and financial difficulties, which are looked at separately in this chapter (see page 79).

One of the difficulties of giving up work, whether you're the managing director of a multinational company or you work two mornings a week for a small local business, is a loss of identity. We all have different roles in life: the roles that we play within our personal life – spouse, parent, son or daughter, brother or sister, friend – and the roles that we play in our working life – employer, employee, colleague. Sadly, many of us tend to undervalue the roles that we play within our families, only recognizing what we do at work as real achievement, which is why we value our working identities so highly. Giving up work, therefore, can not only seem like the end of 'productive' or 'useful' life, it can also seem like the end of a part of yourself – the person that you are at work, you feel, no longer exists. If this happens, it's quite natural to feel a sense of grief at this loss. However, there are plenty of steps that you can take to help yourself through this difficult time.

Although you may have worked for the same company for many years, you may well have been married to your spouse for even longer; you've been a son or daughter all your life, and you've been a parent all your children's lives. These relationships are dear to us, and yet we often put them second after our jobs. If we are successful at work, we feel successful in life, yet we don't seem to see the successful fulfilment of our personal relationships as any sort of achievement. Our loved ones, however, often think differently. Many people who feel that their life is no longer worthwhile will be surprised to hear themselves described as 'wonderful' partners, 'loving and supportive' parents, 'warm and generous' friends. The chances are that the roles that you play in your personal life are in themselves an achievement, so try to recognize that. You may also wish to celebrate the fact that giving up work, while it is undoubtedly a loss of sorts, is also a gain in that you will now have more time to enjoy those relationships; this is particularly valuable if you feel you may have neglected them in the past.

Boredom can be a problem when you give up your job but, in reality, it's likely to be less so than you expect – ask people who have dreaded retirement only to find that, after six months, they wonder how they ever found the time to go to work. You may find it irritating when people say 'take up a hobby', especially as they tend to be rather vague about what such a thing might be. Unless you've already dabbled in the building of ships out of spent matches or the intricate tying of knots to make clever hanging plant holders, the chances are you'll have no desire to start now. One of the problems is that the words 'hobby' and 'pastime' often appear together, giving the impression that a hobby is something you do simply to while away the hours, to 'pass time'. Of course a hobby can have that function, but it can also be stimulating and productive as well as enjoyable. It can give you new skills, new friends and a sense of achievement.

Obviously, the severity of your heart failure will have some bearing on what sort of things you can do with your newly acquired free time. If your symptoms mean that you are unable to go to work, anything that is physically strenuous will be out of the question. If you become breathless easily, you probably won't be able to take up playing the trumpet, although haven't you always wanted to learn the guitar or piano? Painting, creative writing, jewellery-making, genealogy – these are all things that you can do at classes or at home. If you are able to get to your local continuing education centre, you could learn a language, study literature, history, politics – the possibilities are virtually endless. In addition to actually 'taking up' something, don't forget the simple daily pleasures that were always rushed when you had to go to work, things such as walking the dog, having coffee with a friend or taking a leisurely lunch with your family. If your symptoms permit, a little light gardening, decorating or DIY might be all right – check with your doctor, though, and stop if you get unusually breathless.

Financial hardship and claiming benefits

Giving up work is almost certainly going to affect your financial situation. You may also find it difficult to meet the cost of travel to your medical appointments and the cost of prescription charges. If your partner has to take time off work to care for you, or has to give up his or her job as well, then there will be even more impact on your finances.

Whether you have had to give up work or not, there are a number of benefits that you may be able to claim if you are suffering financial hardship as a result of your ill health. These include:

- Disability living allowance – you may be eligible for this allowance if you're aged between 16 and 64, have needed help for three months because of your illness or disability, and are likely to need help for at least another six months. Needing help can mean help with personal care – eating meals, washing and dressing, using the lavatory and so on, or it can mean help with getting around. If you think you may be entitled to this benefit, don't wait until you've needed help for three months before applying – the sooner you set the wheels in motion, the better. If you are very seriously ill and have a life expectancy of less than six months, special rules apply that mean you should get your benefit very quickly.

- Attendance allowance – if you're aged over 65 when you become ill or disabled and you need help to look after yourself, you may be eligible for this allowance.
- Incapacity benefit – if you're under state pension age and can't work because of your illness, you may be eligible for this benefit if you don't get statutory sick pay or if it has ended. You need to have been under state pension age when you became ill, have paid national insurance contributions, be receiving medical treatment and be unable to work for two days or more out of seven. There are some circumstances in which you can carry out 'permitted work' while claiming this benefit, although this could affect other benefits such as housing benefit.

If you need someone to look after you most of the time, and if you receive an attendance allowance or a disability living allowance, your carer may be able to claim a carer's allowance. This is a taxable benefit for people, often husbands or wives, who care for someone else for 35 hours a week or more. Your own benefit may be affected if your carer gets a carer's allowance, so you need to look at all the options.

Depending on your individual circumstances, there may be other benefits that you can claim, as well as certain reductions or exemptions for things like council tax, vehicle tax and some travel costs. You may also be entitled to help with prescription charges, sight tests and dental treatment. The Department of Health's leaflet *Help with health costs* gives more details. Contact the Health Literature Line (see page 106) to order a copy.

All this may seem rather complicated and bewildering, especially when you're also trying to cope with the effects of your heart failure and keep stress to a minimum. Don't be afraid to ask for help. There are people out there whose job it is to make sure you get the support you need, whether it's financial assistance or access to various services that will make your life easier. Talk to the hospital social worker, or ask to speak to a social worker at your local social services department (you'll find the number in Yellow Pages). Your local Citizens Advice Bureau (see page 106) will be able to offer information and advice on coping with debt and applying for financial assistance; they'll also help you fill in those rather alarming forms. For general information and advice on benefits, call the Benefit Enquiry Line (see page 105). Most importantly, try not to worry. It may be a difficult time, but there is lots of support available to help you get through it.

Tips for coping with changes

Some tips for coping with the changes in your life:

- Try to focus on the positive – for example, giving up work may mean more time and closer relationships with your partner, friends, children and grandchildren.
- Focus on what you can do rather than what you can't, and try to accept that you may not be able to do all that you'd like to do
- Adapt your activities so that you can still join in with family and friends, even though it may be in a less active role.
- Take an active role in your treatment – by learning as much as you can about heart failure and its treatment, you'll feel more in control of the situation and you'll be able to work with the medical staff as part of a team.
- Include your partner or carer in your discussions about your condition.
- Keep talking to your partner, family and friends about how you feel about your condition, and about how they feel – it affects them too, because they are the people who love you.
- Consider joining a heart support group (see British Heart Foundation, page 106) where you'll be able to talk to people in a similar position.

9
Sex and relationships

Having a heart problem is bound to affect your relationships with those close to you, especially your relationship with your partner, who will to some extent have become your 'carer'. This may be on a temporary basis while your treatment is sorting itself out, for example; or it may be a more permanent situation. Even if your heart failure is fairly mild and your symptoms are under control, the very fact that there has been some damage to your heart can be quite frightening, which can in itself have an impact on your relationship and in particular your sex life. This can seem the least of your worries when you're first learning to come to terms with a heart problem, but if you usually enjoy a reasonably healthy sex life, resuming it will become more important as you gradually bring your symptoms under control and return to a more normal daily life.

Is it safe to have sex?

If your heart failure isn't severe, there's no reason why you shouldn't resume normal sexual activity as soon as your symptoms are under control. It's quite natural to have some reservations about having sex again, especially if your heart failure is the result of a heart attack. Many couples worry that sex will actually trigger a heart attack but in reality this doesn't ever happen. For most people with heart problems, having sex is like any other form of exercise, and can actually be good for you. But just as you would be sensible to take certain precautions when doing other kinds of exercise, you may feel happier following guidelines suggested for lovemaking:

* Avoid heavy meals for at least two hours before having sex.
* Avoid alcohol for at least three hours before having sex.
* Keep the bedroom warm and make sure the bedding isn't too cold.
* Choose a calm, relaxed setting that's free from interruptions.
* Make sure you're in a comfortable position, possibly with your partner taking a more active role.

9

Sex and relationships

Having a heart problem is bound to affect your relationships with those close to you, especially your relationship with your partner, who will, to some extent, have become your 'carer'. This may be on a temporary basis (while your treatment is kicking in, for example), or it may be a more permanent situation. Even if your heart failure is fairly mild and your symptoms are under control, the very fact that there has been some damage to your heart can be quite frightening, which can in itself have an impact on your relationship and in particular, your sex life. This can seem the least of your worries when you're first coming to terms with a heart problem, but if you usually enjoy a reasonably healthy sex life, resuming it will become more important as you gradually bring your symptoms under control and return to a more normal daily life.

Is it safe to have sex?

If your heart failure isn't severe, there's no reason why you shouldn't resume normal sexual activity as soon as your symptoms are under control. It's quite natural to have some reservations about having sex again, especially if your heart failure is the result of a heart attack. Many couples worry that sex will actually bring on a heart attack but in reality this hardly ever happens. For most people with heart problems, having sex is like any other form of exercise and can actually be good for you. But just as it would be sensible to take certain precautions when doing other forms of exercise, you may feel happier following guidelines suggested for heart patients:

- Avoid heavy meals for at least two hours before having sex.
- Avoid alcohol for at least three hours before having sex.
- Keep the bedroom warm and make sure the bedding isn't too cold.
- Choose a calm, relaxed setting that's free from interruptions.
- Make sure you're in a comfortable position, possibly with your partner taking a more active role.

- Stop and rest if you feel unreasonably breathless, uncomfortable or tired.

It's important to remember that, even if you're feeling physically well, you may not feel ready to resume your sex life right away. This is perfectly normal, and in many cases, your desire to have sex will return naturally as you gradually learn to cope with your heart failure. In some cases, however, sexual feelings do not return of their own accord; in others, the desire returns but a physical problem prevents you from expressing it. This can be very frustrating, but fear not – there is plenty that can be done to help.

Erectile dysfunction

Erectile dysfunction or impotence is when a man has difficulty getting an erection that's strong enough, or when he gets an erection but has trouble maintaining it. This is a problem experienced by at least one man in 10, and it is fairly common in men with heart problems. There are a number of possible causes, which may be physical or psychological, or a combination of both.

As we have already seen, many people with heart failure have narrowed arteries, and if the blood vessels that lead to the penis are furred up, it's likely that the blood supply is insufficient to achieve or maintain an erection. In fact, some doctors see impotence as a possible symptom of heart disease even if their patient isn't aware of any heart problems at the time. A study in Texas involving 8,000 men found a significant link between erectile dysfunction and increased risk of heart disease. The research concluded that no patient should be treated for impotence without the possibility of cardiovascular disease being investigated. Similarly, because many people are too embarrassed to start talking about sexual difficulties, doctors treating patients for heart problems should mention erectile dysfunction as a possible complication of heart disease.

Erectile dysfunction is even more likely in smokers because nicotine causes the blood vessels to constrict, reducing blood flow to the penis. Yet another reason to ditch the filthy weed – as if you needed another reason!

Some types of heart medication, especially some beta-blockers and blood pressure drugs, may cause erection problems and may also affect your ability to have an orgasm. Some types of antidepressants can have a similar effect and can also cause loss of libido. If you think the problems you're having may be due to the side effects of the medicines you're taking, talk to your doctor or heart failure nurse – if they don't know you're having problems, they won't be able to help. The solution may be as simple as changing to a different type of medication.

There may also be a psychological or emotional reason that you're having problems getting an erection. If the problem has only started since you became ill, it's quite likely to be linked to your feelings about your condition. Even if your symptoms are well controlled, simply knowing that you have a chronic condition can be very stressful, and negative stress can affect your ability to achieve an erection and your libido in general.

Loss of libido

Both men and women can experience a lessening or a complete loss of sexual desire as a consequence of their heart problems. This may be due to feeling physically unwell, or it could be a result of stress, anxiety and depression, all of which are natural reactions to learning that you have heart failure. Also, simply knowing that you have an incurable condition can change the way you view yourself, and this too can lead to a loss of sexual desire. This is often a temporary situation, but if it happens to you, whether the cause is physical or psychological, it's important to address it fairly quickly so that it doesn't become more of a problem than it needs to be.

What can be done?

The good news is that there are a number of things that can be done to improve the situation. The two most important things to remember are: first, you should not be embarrassed about discussing sexual problems with your doctor or heart failure nurse – most of us experience some type of sexual problem at some point in our lives, and your doctor or nurse really will have heard it all before; and second, and even more important, you should discuss the issue with your partner. Whatever the root cause of the problem, it is a problem for the couple, not just for one partner. If there's a physical aspect, it may be that you need to change your medication, start taking a new medicine or use a medical device. But even though it's you that needs to take action, you should discuss everything with your partner; after all, your sexual relationship is something you have created and nurtured between you, and any problems with it should have the attention and tender loving care of both partners. If you find it difficult to discuss your sexual relationship, try to get comfortable with the topic first by discussing sex in a more general way, perhaps after watching a television programme or reading a magazine article. Once you're used to doing this, it will be easier to talk about what's happening in your own sex lives.

Treatment for erectile dysfunction

The best starting point in dealing with erection problems is probably your GP, and it's best if you and your partner attend together, booking a double appointment, if possible, so that you don't feel rushed. Your doctor may be able to offer advice, suggest a change in any medication you're already taking or prescribe a new drug to help the problem.

You will have almost certainly heard of Viagra, which is the brand name of a drug called sildenafil, the first phosphodiesterase type-5 (PDE-5) inhibitor, which came on the market in 1998. There are now two other PDE-5 inhibitors available: tadafil (brand name: Cialis) and vardenafil (brand name: Levitra). These drugs increase the body's ability to achieve and maintain an erection, and you take them about 30 minutes before you have sex. Not everyone with heart failure will be able to take PDE-5 inhibitors though, either because of the condition itself or because of possible interactions with other drugs, especially blood pressure medications. Your doctor or specialist will need to do a thorough assessment and go through with you all the other pills or medicines you're taking, including those that are not on prescription.

Other treatments for erectile dysfunction include injections into the penis (not as bad as it sounds) and vacuum pumps. Your doctor will be able to advise you on the suitability of these treatments. Alternatively, he or she may refer you to a specialist clinic where the doctors have particular expertise in sexual difficulties.

If no underlying physical cause can be found, you might want to consider consulting a psychosexual counsellor or therapist. Relate, the best known organization for relationship counselling, now offers help for sexual problems and has a number of trained psychosexual therapists. Relate usually makes a small charge for its services, based closely on what you can afford. If you have access to the internet, Relate also offers online help with sexual problems. This is a tempting option if you find it embarrassing to talk about the difficulties, but do remember that all their therapists are highly trained and have seen and heard it all before.

You may have to wait a while for an appointment, but don't put your sex life on hold until you've seen the right doctor or therapist or until you've taken the right pills. There is plenty you can do to keep things going while you're waiting. If you have erection problems but still have a healthy libido, forget about penetrative sex for a while and go back to the things you used to do when you first met, before you went 'all the way'. When we settle into long, comfortable loving relationships, many of us are inclined to become sexually lazy. We know how our partner's body works and we know exactly how to have enjoyable and satisfying intercourse; as a result, we tend to skimp on the other types of sexual contact which, when you think about it, is a great shame. Think back to when you were young and just embarking on your first sexual relationships. Remember how inventive you could be when you knew your parents were only in the next room? Now's your chance to rekindle the excitement and add a new dimension to your sex life in the process.

Intimacy

If either or both of you have temporarily gone off sex, don't worry: there's no law that says you must have intercourse however many times a week or month. Try to think instead about intimacy. Intimacy is important to both partners throughout a relationship, and it's even more so when sexual activity is not possible, either permanently or temporarily.

If you possibly can, try to maintain some physical contact, even if it's only the odd kiss or cuddle during the course of your day. Simply holding hands or snuggling up together on the sofa can be very reassuring and nourishing for a relationship where sex is 'on hold'. And if you can maintain some contact, it'll be easier to resume your sexual relationship once you are ready.

If you don't feel ready for any sexual contact, it may be a good idea to set boundaries when you touch each other. Talk to your partner, and be clear about no-go areas so that you can avoid 'mixed signals'. Where there is no physical cause for erectile difficulty or loss of libido, you may even find that restrictions on your bedtime activity actually stimulate desire. It's widely acknowledged in these cases that banning sexual contact for a while can help a man to get erections again – it removes the pressure to 'perform', thus relieving stress and anxiety that may have been contributing to the problem. Also, it seems to be human nature to want what we can't have!

It's vital to talk with your partner about what's happening in your sexual relationship and what bearing you feel your heart failure may have on things. In many cases, a temporary physical problem leads to a longer-term psychological one: a man has trouble getting an erection so he finds himself avoiding sexual contact; this makes his partner think he's not interested, causing her to stop initiating sex, which in turn leads to him thinking she no longer finds him attractive. It's the same for a woman: if she's nervous, she may find it difficult to relax enough to become sufficiently aroused. This can make penetration painful, which leads her to avoid sex, making her partner think she's gone off him. And so on, and so on – it's a vicious circle.

By openly discussing the issue, you'll be creating more intimacy, and this in itself can go some way to healing problems with the loss of confidence that is so closely linked with impotence and loss of libido. Simply talking about and focusing on sex can stimulate interest and desire, but if you do decide you need outside help, you'll have already done some of the groundwork by discussing the problems with your partner, and it can be hoped that you'll both be relaxed and comfortable with each other and ready to tackle the problem together.

10

Caring for someone with heart failure

The text in this chapter often refers to the person with heart failure as 'your partner', but this is not intended to exclude those caring for a parent, other relative or friend; the term is used here for simplicity, and most of the information will be of use to all those caring for a loved one with heart failure.

If you have to look after a relative or friend because heart failure means he or she can't manage on his or her own, even if the situation is temporary, you are technically that person's carer. You're not alone – there are an estimated seven million carers in the UK. That's around one in seven adults who look after someone, often their partner, because of an illness or disability. Being a carer can be physically and emotionally exhausting, not to mention frightening. You may still be feeling very shocked at your loved one's diagnosis and you'll naturally be very worried about your partner's condition and how it's likely to progress. Added to that, you have the extra burden of trying to reassure your partner, and of trying to take in and understand everything the doctors are saying. It's quite likely that neither of you will take very much in at first, but in the few days and weeks following the diagnosis, you should find things a little easier. It's also likely that you'll feel overwhelmed by the responsibility at first, but this too will settle down as you become more informed about what your new role involves and what help is available.

Understanding the condition

The more clearly you understand your partner's condition, the more you will be able to help him or her. It will also be less frightening for you if you understand exactly what is happening, both in terms of the condition itself and in terms of the various tests and treatments that may be carried out. Chapters 1 and 2 will help you to understand what heart failure is and what the possible causes may be, and Chapters 3, 4 and 5 look at testing and treatment. You will probably have some questions that apply specifically to your partner's case, so you'll need to talk to the GP, specialist or heart failure nurse about these. It might be an idea to jot down the questions before your appointment, because it can be very difficult to remember everything you wanted to ask, especially when you're feeling worried or anxious. The sort of things you might want to ask are things such as:

- What drugs should my partner be taking, how much, when and how often?
- Are there any serious side effects we should watch for, and what should we do if these occur?
- Will my partner need surgery? When will this happen and how do we prepare?
- What sort of physical activity is best? When and for how long?
- What sort of diet should my partner be eating?
- What else can I do to help my partner?
- What help is available from the hospital, the community health team or the local authority?

Asking questions while you're at the hospital can be daunting, especially when everyone looks so busy. Try saying, 'I have some questions about my partner's condition and treatment. Who is it best to talk to and when would be a convenient time?' This gives them the opportunity to arrange a time that will suit them so that they can answer your questions fully and in an unhurried manner.

How you may react to your partner's illness

In the first few days and even weeks after the diagnosis, you are likely to go through a number of emotions, some of which will be similar to those experienced by your partner, such as anger, sadness and even guilt. You may also feel a sense of resentment. (Then you feel guilty about that, too!)

These are all perfectly normal and understandable reactions to something major that's happened in your lives. The fact that they're normal reactions probably doesn't help much, does it? So try to think about what, if anything, you can do about them.

Anger

You may feel angry in the sense of 'why did this have to happen?' or 'why us?', especially if your partner has had a fairly healthy lifestyle or seems too young to have a heart problem. Your partner may feel this way as well, and it's something the two of you can talk about together. Don't worry about saying 'it's not fair', because you're right – it isn't fair! But it is something that has happened and what you need to do now – after allowing yourselves a little 'moaning time' – is find the best way to deal with it. It can be immensely comforting to discuss this together and to make plans for how you're going to cope. On the other hand, you may actually feel angry with your partner for becoming ill, especially if you've been on at them for some time to give up smoking or cut down on alcohol or eat more healthily, and so on and so forth. Again, this is normal and understandable, but unfortunately, whether your partner's lifestyle contributed to the heart failure or not, the situation cannot be reversed and the important thing now is to find a way to improve matters from now on. Don't allow the anger to build or it might flare up one day and result in bad feeling between you, and you have enough to cope with at the moment without having a big bust-up with your other half. It might help to talk to your partner about how you feel if you can do so without letting things get out of hand. You could say something like, 'I love you very much, but I feel quite angry with you at the moment because I believe your smoking has contributed to your illness, and the fact that you're ill makes me very sad.' Simply getting it off your chest can make you feel better, and your partner will understand that your anger stems from love. If it's not possible to discuss it with your partner, try to talk it through with someone who understands – another carer, perhaps, or a trained counsellor. This should help you put your anger into the background so that it becomes easier to deal with. Another thing you could try is writing down exactly how you feel – have a really good rant – then tear up the paper and throw it away, or if you're typing on a keyboard, simply delete the words. If you know that what you've written is not going to be read ever again, you can pour all that anger out and feel quite cleansed as a result. People who try this often say they feel a great weight has been lifted afterwards.

Sadness

Sadness is best dealt with in a similar way to the 'why us?' type of anger. Talk to each other about how you feel; moan, commiserate, accept that you have a right to feel sad, cry if you want to. It doesn't matter if you do this a few times, but try to include some positive notes each time you talk. It can be hoped that your partner's symptoms will be brought swiftly under control and that you can both look forward to getting back to normal fairly soon. If your partner's heart failure is more severe, finding something to look forward to might seem difficult, but give it a try. One positive thing is that, now that the heart failure has been diagnosed, treatment can begin, which means that the symptoms should start to improve.

Both you and your partner are likely to feel sad or low from time to time, and you'll probably get used to having good days and bad days. Sometimes, however, these feelings are overwhelming and long-lasting, and if you feel unable to pull yourself out of a low mood, or if feelings of sadness turn to feelings of despair and hopelessness, you may be suffering from depression (see page 68). There are several ways of dealing with this depending on your own history and circumstances, but talk to your doctor first, as he or she will be able to point you in the right direction.

Guilt

Again, guilt is something you're both likely to feel – your partner may feel guilty for not stopping smoking, for drinking too much, for eating too many fry-ups and so on. At the same time, you blame yourself – why didn't you stop your partner from smoking and drinking? Why didn't you make sure that he or she ate healthily, took more exercise and so on? The thing is, there will always be something you can blame yourself for, and unless you strapped your partner down and force-fed him or her pies and chips washed down with brandy and followed by a couple of cigarettes, that blame is unreasonable. It's true that an unhealthy lifestyle may contribute to the problems that cause heart failure, but it's also true that, even if your partner's diet and lifestyle had been healthier, the heart failure might still have developed. The important thing now is to look at what you can do to improve matters in the future, not what you did that might – and only 'might'– have made a difference in the past.

Resentment

Most people who find themselves caring for someone who is ill feel resentment at some point. It's hardly surprising, when you think about it – you will have had to make significant changes to your life because of your partner's heart failure. These changes could include having to give up your job, having to take more (or complete) responsibility for running the household, being unable to see your friends as much as usual and having less time for yourself in general. In addition, of course, you'll be spending a considerable amount of time on your partner's illness. Depending on how severe the heart failure is, this could range from simply accompanying your partner to hospital appointments to helping with washing, dressing and moving about the house.

Not only that, but you may find your partner more 'difficult' than usual. He or she may seem irritable, moody and self-obsessed – all natural responses to having a heart condition and probably feeling quite poorly. Worse still, you may feel that your partner is ungrateful and doesn't appreciate your sacrifices. Don't feel guilty for feeling this way – there's not a carer in the country who hasn't at some point felt like yelling at his or her partner, smashing a few plates and walking out. The trick is to try and let off steam in other ways so that you don't take it out on your partner – or anyone else in the family for that matter.

Talk to your partner about your feelings if you possibly can. Choose your time carefully, though. It's better to talk about difficult feelings when you're both feeling reasonably calm – if your partner snaps at you for no reason, don't snap back. Wait until your partner seem more relaxed and say something like, 'I know that feeling weak and breathless all the time must really be getting you down, but when you snap at me like you did earlier, I find it very upsetting.'

If you feel you can't talk to your partner, make time to phone a friend or, ideally, someone who is in a similar situation. There are a number of support networks for carers (see page 108), and it's worth looking into these because sometimes you really need to talk to someone who knows exactly what you're going through.

Will your relationship change?

Some change in your relationship is inevitable, but it doesn't have to be a negative change and, in fact, many couples find they become closer through the experience. Things will obviously be different for a while – you may be taking on roles that your partner has always taken up until now, and it can take a while for you both to adjust to this. But it becomes easier if you keep talking to each other about these changes and how you feel about them.

Where there is a negative change in a couple's relationship, it tends to occur when the feelings of anger, guilt and resentment discussed above have been allowed to build up and fester. The importance of talking about what's happening really can't be stressed enough. Try to look at discussion as 'relationship protection' – it doesn't make the illness go away, but it keeps the connection between the two of you alive and it helps to keep you on the same side.

We've looked at the possible changes in your partner's personality – your partner may have become more irritable, moody or whatever – but you may not have noticed how you yourself have changed in response to your partner's condition. For example, you may feel exactly the same as your partner in many ways – angry, sad and so on – but because you're not the one with the illness, you may feel you have to put on a brave face and stay cheerful. Keeping your frustrations bottled up can be a tremendous strain, causing stress or even leading to depression. You may also find yourself becoming overprotective and even obsessed with your partner's condition. Of course you're worried about your loved one, and of course you want to make sure that your partner doesn't do anything that's going to cause further damage to the heart or make the symptoms worse. But you must be careful not to make your partner feel more ill than he or she actually is, or to remove all feelings of independence. You may find that you're trying to protect your partner from stress and worry, and while you're clearly doing this for the best possible reasons, it may not be the best thing for your partner, or for you. If you try to deal with all the day-to-day worries in life on your own – domestic worries, bills, family problems and so on – you'll begin to feel overburdened and your partner will feel excluded, and that won't do either of you any good. Talk about these issues as they occur; try to make decisions and solve problems *together*.

It's important that people who have been ill with heart failure should regain their independence and get back to normal as soon as possible. Let your partner decide how much he or she is ready to take on, whether this is in terms of physical activity – a gentle exercise programme is often beneficial – or in terms of general involvement in family life.

Sexual problems

Sexual problems as a result of heart failure can often be fairly easily overcome, but if one or both partners feel embarrassed and reluctant to discuss the situation, it can be more difficult to deal with, so it really is best to address it as soon as possible.

It's quite common for the partners of people with heart failure to be nervous about resuming sexual activity because they are worried that this will put a strain on their partner's heart or will make their heart failure symptoms worse. In most cases, these worries are unfounded, but if you're in any doubt at all, have a chat with your doctor or the heart failure nurse. There are some guidelines for heart patients (see page 83) and you might find it reassuring to follow these, especially at first.

Another common problem can be a temporary loss of attraction. When one partner is ill and the other takes the role of carer, it can sometimes be difficult to maintain your view of one another as sexual people, and this can lead to physical problems and lack of desire. Don't worry if neither of you feel like sex for a while – coping with heart failure can be exhausting for both of you – but once the symptoms are under control you should be able to start gradually returning to normal. In the mean time, try to keep things 'ticking over' by making sure you have plenty of physical contact, even if it's not sexual. Holding hands, sitting close to one another, kissing and cuddling are all ways of demonstrating affection and closeness without necessarily going on to have sex.

If there are physical difficulties such as erection problems, these may be due to side effects of your partner's heart failure medicine. Your doctor may be able to adjust the medication or prescribe another medicine to help the situation. If the problem is lack of desire, you may need to think about how you see one another at the moment – do you see your partner as a dependent, vulnerable, sick person? Does your partner see you as a nurse or parent figure? If this happens – and it often does in this situation – you need to work at becoming a couple again. It might help to set aside some time together and play 'do you remember?' Think back to your early days together: try to recall some of the things you did, the places you went, the films you saw. Think about what attracted you to one another when you first met. Tell your partner how you felt waiting for him or her to turn up for a date, or how you felt when you decided to get married or move in together. Remembering your lives as lovers will help to re-establish those roles in your mind and enable you to build on this to rekindle some of the flutterings of desire that you once took for granted.

You may find it helpful to read through Chapter 9, which, although it is aimed primarily at the person with heart failure, looks at sexual difficulties in a little more detail. Remember, a sexual problem is a problem for the couple, not just for one person, so work on this together, and together you can enjoy the rewards.

Looking after yourself

Caring for someone with heart failure can be a tough, demanding job, and it's one that you may not get much (or any) thanks for, at least for a while. Feeling tired and stressed is not uncommon. Even if you don't have to attend much to your partner's physical needs, simply having to take extra responsibility for domestic and administrative chores can take it out of you.

Diane
Diane, wife of Peter Houghton (see page 45) found one of the most difficult things about her husband's illness was coping with the extra responsibility:

It was the feeling of being the 'one in charge'. Peter was so ill that I found myself having to make all the decisions, and even though some of them were only trivial, domestic things, it felt like a lot to cope with on top of the day-to-day problems of looking after him and worrying about him. His heart failure developed over several years, so fortunately I got used to doing the extra physical work quite slowly, but it was still difficult. Peter couldn't work any more so I became the main breadwinner, which was also a lot of responsibility. My job was quite stressful and demanding – I was a lecturer in English for international students – but I enjoyed it and I think it helped me to cope. There were problems, of course, because I couldn't take time off, and when Peter was in hospital in Oxford, I could only see him twice a week because we lived in

Birmingham. But it gave me something else to focus on and I think that's important. In fact, that's the best advice I have for someone in a similar situation: keep something for yourself – you shouldn't feel guilty for not making your whole life revolve around your partner. You also need to learn to take each day as it comes. Peter is still severely disabled, but his quality of life is so much better than before his operation, and as for me, well, I always say, if he's all right, I'm all right!

It's not uncommon for those caring for a sick partner to end up feeling physically run down and exhausted. You'll probably have spent a considerable amount of time thinking about your partner's diet and pattern of exercise, but how much have you thought about your own health? Being busy all the time may mean you grab a less-than-healthy snack because it's quicker. For the same reason, you don't get enough sleep, you neglect your friends, your hobbies and even other members of the family. All these factors can affect your health, weakening your immune system and making you vulnerable to every bug that's going around. If you find yourself feeling guilty about putting your own needs before those of your partner, try to look at it another way: if you're struck down by flu or whatever because your immune system is weakened, how are you going to be able to care for your partner? And who's going to look after you?

To a certain extent, matters are out of your hands – you cannot take away your partner's heart failure – but there are aspects of caring where you can make changes to make the situation less stressful.

Taking control and reducing stress

Your partner may be affected by stress as a result of his or her heart failure, and this is looked at in some detail in Chapter 8. But it can also be very stressful to care for someone with the condition. Stress can occur as a result of feeling out of control and of trying to do too much in too little time. What makes this even more difficult is that the more incapacitated your partner is by heart failure, the more time he or she will have; you, on the other hand, will have half the time and twice the work you had before. This can be difficult for your partner to understand. Your partner may expect too much of you, want you to sit and chat for long periods of time or to bring drinks and snacks as soon as they are asked for, or send you on countless errands throughout the day. Of course your partner will be bored and will want your company, and if he or she really is physically unable to prepare snacks and drinks, then of course you'll be expected to respond as soon as a cup of tea or whatever is demanded.

This is where you need to take control. It's not that you should refuse these things, but you need to organize a routine and explain to your partner that, while it's nice to take spontaneous breaks, it really isn't possible to do that too often at the moment.

It's important that you do spend some leisure time together, but if you're busy, you need to organize your days more carefully. Maybe you could timetable meals and snacks and plan to sit with your partner for half an hour while you take a mid-morning break. Perhaps you could take a gentle walk together after lunch, and plan another half-hour break with your afternoon tea. Most of us become slightly self-obsessed when we're ill, and your partner may find it difficult to understand why you can't just drop everything the minute you're asked. But if your partner knows that he or she will have your attention (and the sandwich or tea and biscuit or whatever) at specific times during the day, he or she will be reassured and find it easier to fit into your routine. This has the double benefit of ensuring you take adequate breaks – research suggests that regular breaks can make you more productive, so you end up achieving more over the day than if you'd worked right through – and of allowing your partner to feel loved and cared for without disrupting your entire day. If you're able to put this into practice, it ought to reduce stress for both of you.

It's also important for you to make some time for yourself and your own needs. If your usual routine involves an evening class once a week, a round of golf on Sunday and seeing friends for coffee or the odd night out, and then you suddenly find you're not doing any of those things, resentment is likely to build up. It may be the case that things have to go on hold for a while if your partner is very ill, but once the symptoms are under control, things should improve, and you should be able to pick up some of your usual activities. If your partner really is too ill to be left alone, arrange for another relative or friend to come and sit while you go out. You should not feel guilty about taking some time out for yourself – you will be a better carer if you have some time off from focusing on your partner's needs. It can also be helpful for your partner, who may be well aware of the sacrifices you have had to make in order to care for him or her.

Bill

Bill, aged 63, was diagnosed with heart failure two years ago, having previously suffered two heart attacks. His wife Eileen was so worried about him that she was reluctant to leave him even while she went shopping. Bill remembers:

I was very poorly at first, and I could barely walk around the house, but now I take lots of different pills and potions and, though I don't expect I'll be running the marathon, I'm much better. I had to take it easy at first – I couldn't get up and down the stairs so we got a bed made up in the front room and I slept in there for about four months. Eileen was absolutely marvellous. Fortunately, she'd just retired, so there weren't any problems with work, but she completely gave up a very busy social life to look after me when I came out of hospital. I know she was worried that if I did things for myself, I'd put a strain on my heart and make my heart failure worse. I assured her I'd be careful, but even though I nagged her, she didn't want to leave me. In the end, it was the heart failure nurse who managed to convince her that I'd be fine on my own. Now she's back going to all her classes again and I'm really pleased. She's happier to be seeing her friends and doing her various hobbies and I get to watch the footie or the snooker on the telly in peace!

Healthy eating

You'll want to make sure that your partner has the best possible diet to ensure that his or her heart stays as healthy as possible from now on. Ways of having a 'heart-friendly' diet are covered in depth in Chapter 6. If you follow roughly the same diet as your partner, not only will you be reducing your own risk of developing coronary heart disease (and other conditions such as diabetes) in the future, but you'll start to feel fitter and healthier in general.

Eating healthily is all the more important when you're caring for someone else because of the extra demands you're putting on your own body. Eating more fruit and vegetables, preferably raw or very lightly cooked, and less sugar and saturated fat will help to keep your immune system working properly and will make you feel more alert and energized. Make sure you don't skip meals because you're busy. If you don't fancy a big meal, just have smaller portions and eat more frequently – some experts say that 'little and often' is better for the digestion anyway. If you find yourself skipping breakfast you'll start to feel hungry or tired by mid- or late morning, and that's when you're likely to grab a sugary snack such as biscuits or chocolate to keep you going. It's true that these foods will give you a temporary energy boost, but it really is only temporary, and as your blood sugar levels rise sharply and then fall again, you're likely to experience an 'energy slump'. Try to eat a good breakfast that will keep you going until lunchtime. If you do start to feel hungry mid-morning, have some fruit, a couple of savoury biscuits or a semi-sweet biscuit. If you don't want, or need (for health reasons), to follow exactly the same diet as your partner, just try to follow these basic guidelines:

- Eat more fruit and vegetables. Aim for two or three pieces of fruit a day and three or four portions of vegetables – salads, vegetable soups and vegetable juices all count towards your total.
- Cut down on sugary foods such as sweets, cakes and biscuits.
- Cut down on salt, especially if you have high blood pressure.
- Eat less saturated (animal) fats – replace butter or margarine with olive oil-based spread or low-fat spread.
- Avoid 'ready meals' and takeaways.
- Choose lean cuts of meat and poultry (with the skin removed) and oily fish such as salmon, trout, mackerel, herring and sardines.
- Cook with olive oil instead of butter or lard.
- Remember you are what you eat – are you a bright, shiny crisp apple? Or a fat, stodgy, greasy doughnut?

When the going gets tough

There are bound to be times when you feel isolated by your situation or even that you can't cope. This is quite likely to happen if your partner is very dependent but not ill enough to be in hospital, but it can also happen when you've been caring at a fairly low level for a long time. Even if your partner doesn't need help with dressing and feeding and getting around, it could just be that he or she is depressed by the illness and needs a lot of your attention. Sometimes people with an ongoing condition like heart failure appear to have undergone a personality change and can be quite grumpy or irritable with those around them. Or maybe it's simply that your partner can no longer work or go out very much and you just feel you never have any time alone.

Talking to friends or other family members can help when you feel like this, but sometimes it can be more useful to talk to someone who is in a similar situation and really understands what you're going through. Talk to the heart failure nurse or the practice nurse at your doctor's surgery – they should be able to tell you if there is a carers' or heart support group (for people with heart problems and their families) in your area. Or you can contact the British Heart Foundation (see page 106), who keep an up-to-date list of all the heart support groups linked to their organization in England and Wales.

If you have access to the internet, support is available through various online networks such as that run by the Princess Royal Trust for Carers (see page 108). There are also organizations that offer telephone support for those unable to attend group meetings. The British Cardiac Patients Association, for example, offers support and information to patients and carers via meetings, telephone, fax or email (see page 105).

Practical help with caring

People with heart failure can become incapacitated by their condition, especially if they also have other health problems or are becoming frail because of advancing age. If the person you're looking after requires a high level of care or a lot of attention, you may need more than emotional support, and you shouldn't wait until you're exhausted or simply can't cope any more before you ask for help. There are a number of organizations that may be able to help, often with no charge. A good starting point is your local social services department (listed in the phone book under 'local authority'), who will be able to organize a carer's assessment for you. This assessment will look at the sort of care the person you're caring for needs, what help you are providing at the moment and how that is affecting your own life and health. The social services department will use the assessment to decide what can be offered to you. This may include things like providing equipment or a grant to adapt your home – for example, the fitting of handrails, or ramps for a wheelchair. You may be able to get help at home, perhaps with getting your partner washed and dressed, preparing meals or doing the housework.

As we've seen, people with heart failure can become quite bad-tempered with their carers, probably because they feel frustrated at not being able to do things for themselves. You may find that the person you care for is reluctant to accept outside help; this is probably because to do so would be to accept that the condition is debilitating, and that may be difficult to face. Try to keep talking calmly about the situation, explaining that you need some help and that both your lives will be improved as a result. Most people accept this eventually, but in the mean time, the social services department may be able to support you in other ways, so it's still worth getting in touch with them.

Respite care

Every carer needs a break sometimes, and if your partner can't be left and there's no one else to take over for a while, you may be able to organize some 'respite care'. This is where someone else looks after your partner for a time while you have a break. This might be in the home, where a trained carer stays with your partner while you see friends, catch up on your reading or even just have a bath or a few hours' extra sleep. Or it might be that residential respite care is more appropriate. You may need a longer break for a number of reasons – maybe you want to visit your grandchildren, go to a family wedding or have a holiday without your partner. Don't feel guilty about this – you'll be able to cope better if you have a chance to recharge your batteries. Or maybe you're ill yourself, or you need to go into hospital for a routine procedure.

Respite services are provided by a range of organizations such as social services, health authorities, voluntary organizations and private agencies. In many cases, these services will be free or the organization may make a minimal charge. Contact details for some of these organizations can be found in the Useful addresses section (pages 105–9).

Looking to the future

As we've seen, heart failure cannot be cured as such, but there are many treatments to improve the condition, including medicines, surgery and non-surgical procedures along with self-help strategies like the sort of changes in diet and lifestyle that are discussed in this book. With the modern treatments available, together with what we now know about how people with the condition can help their own recovery, many people with heart failure will return to daily life with renewed enthusiasm for living a healthier, more fulfilled life, often for many years to come.

Useful addresses

Age Concern
Astral House
1268 London Road
London SW16 4ER
Helpline: 0800 00 99 66
Website: www.ageconcern.org.uk
Many useful fact sheets available.

American Heart Association
National Center
7272 Greenville Avenue
Dallas, TX 75231
Website: www.americanheart.org

Benefit Enquiry Line
Victoria House
9th Floor
Ormskirk Road
Preston
Lancashire PR1 2QP
Tel.: 0800 88 22 00

British Cardiac Patients Association
Unit 5D
2 Station Road
Swavesey
Cambridge CB4 5QJ
Tel.: 01954 202022
National Helpline: 01223 846845
Website: www.bcpa.co.uk
Email: enquiries@bcpa.co.uk

British Heart Foundation
14 Fitzhardinge Street
London W1H 4DH
Tel.: 020 7935 0185
Heart Information Line: 08450 70 80 70 (9 a.m. to 5 p.m., Monday to Friday)
For list of heart support groups: 020 7487 7110
Website: www.bhf.org.uk

Citizens Advice Bureau (CAB)
Tel.: 020 7833 2181 (admin only)
Website: www.citizensadvice.org.uk

Crossroads Association
10 Regent Place
Rugby
Warwickshire CV21 2PN
Tel.: 0845 450 0350
Website: www.crossroads.org.uk
To arrange respite care for carers.

Cruse Bereavement Care
Cruse House
126 Sheen Road
Richmond
Surrey TW9 1UR
Helpline: 0870 167 1677
Young Persons' Helpline: Freephone 0808 808 1677
Website: www.crusebereavementcare.org.uk

Department of Health
Health Literature Line: 0800 555 777

ExtraLife Limited
The Manor Hospital
Beech Road
Headington
Oxford OX3 7RP
Tel.: 01865 307 583
Website: www.extralife.org.uk
For information on privately funded advanced cardiac techniques.

Heart Failure Foundation
Peter Houghton, c/o Stephen Westaby
Department of Cardiac Surgery
Level 1, John Radcliffe Hospital
Headley Way, Headington
Oxford OX3 9DU
Tel.: (Mr Westaby's secretary) 01865 220269
Website: www.ahf.org.uk

Heart Link
25 Close Street
Hemsworth
Pontefract
West Yorkshire WF9 4QP
Tel.: 01977 613858
Website: www.heartlink.org.uk

H-E-A-R-T UK
7 North Road
Maidenhead
Berkshire SL6 1PE
Tel.: 01628 628 638
Website: www.heartuk.org.uk
Email: ask@heartuk.org.uk

If I Should Die.co.uk
This website was created to provide general information on death
and bereavement without being linked to a particular religion,
philosophy or 'angle' such as financial planning.
Website: www.ifishoulddie.co.uk

International Stress Management Association
PO Box 26
South Petherton TA13 5WY
Tel.: 07000 780430
Website: www.isma.org.uk

National Debtline
Tel.: 0808 808 4000
Website: www.nationaldebtline.co.uk

National Heart Forum
Entrance D, Tavistock House South
Tavistock Square
London WC1H 9LG
Tel.: 020 7383 7638
Website: www.heartforum.org.uk
UK alliance of national organizations working to prevent coronary
heart disease.

NHS Direct
Tel.: 0845 46 47
Website: www.nhsdirect.nhs.uk

Princess Royal Trust for Carers (London office)
142 Minories
London EC3N 1LB
Tel.: 020 7480 7788
Website: www.carers.org

Princess Royal Trust for Carers (Northern office)
Suite 4
Oak House
High Street
Chorley PR7 1DW
Tel.: 01257 234070
Website: www.carers.org
Offices also for Wales and Scotland: contact details provided on
website.

UK Transplant
Communications Directorate
Fox Den Road
Stoke Gifford
Bristol BS34 8RR
Tel.: 0117 975 7575

Organ Donor Line: 0845 60 60 400
Website: www.uktransplant.org.uk

Weight Watchers
Look in the phone book for local groups, or log on to:
www.weightwatchers.co.uk

Further reading

Battison, Toni. *Caring for someone with a heart problem.* Age Concern Books, 2004.

British Heart Foundation. *Heart health.* (A free quarterly magazine produced by British Heart Foundation.)

Cantopher, Tim. *Depressive illness, the curse of the strong.* Sheldon Press, 2003.

Carr, Allen. *Allen Carr's Easy Way to Stop Smoking.* Penguin Books Ltd, 2006.

Cowie, Martin R. *Living with heart failure: a guide for patients.* Bladon Medical Publishing, 2003.

Dymond, Duncan. *The plain English guide to heart disease.* Metro, 2003.

Eckersley, Jill. *Every woman's guide to heart health.* Sheldon Press, 2006.

Gittleman, Ann Louise. *Get the salt out: 501 simple ways to cut salt out of any diet.* Crown Publications, 1997.

Povey, Robert et al. *Eating for a healthy heart.* Sheldon Press, 2005.

Tubbs, Irene. *The heart recovery book.* Sheldon Press, 2006.

Tugendhat, Julia. *How to approach death.* Sheldon Press, forthcoming.

Index